Living with Lupus Nephritis

Living with Lupus Nephritis:

A Comprehensive Guide for Patients

By

Fahad Aziz and Tripti Singh

Cambridge Scholars
Publishing

Living with Lupus Nephritis: A Comprehensive Guide for Patients

By Fahad Aziz and Tripti Singh

With contributions by
Chapter 6: Shivani Garg
Chapter 7: Mansi Jain
Chapter 8: Zohreh Gholizadeh Ghozloujeh, Sayna Norouzi

This book first published 2026

Cambridge Scholars Publishing

Lady Stephenson Library, Newcastle upon Tyne, NE6 2PA, UK

British Library Cataloguing in Publication Data
A catalogue record for this book is available from the British Library

ISBN: 978-1-0364-7398-3
ISBN (Ebook): 978-1-0364-7399-0

TABLE OF CONTENTS

Chapter 1 1
Your Journey with Lupus Nephritis
You are not alone—strength and hope are always within reach.

Chapter 2 9
When Lupus Affects the Kidneys
Understand how lupus changes kidney health.

Chapter 3 26
Early Signs and Symptoms
Learn to recognize the early clues from your body.

Chapter 4 36
How Doctors Detect Lupus Nephritis
See how tests and scans guide diagnosis.

Chapter 5 57
Treatments That Help
Explore options that protect and heal your kidneys.

Chapter 6 92
Your Guide to Medications
Simple steps to stay on track with treatment.
By Shivani Garg MD PhD

Chapter 7 108
Eating for Kidney Health
Nourishing choices that support your body daily.
By Mansi Jain

Chapter 8 126
Pregnancy and Lupus Nephritis
What to know when planning a family with lupus.
By Zohreh Gholizadeh Ghozloujeh and Sayna Norouzi

Chapter 9 140
Managing the Costs of Care
Find ways to ease financial stress of treatment.

Chapter 10 150
Life After Kidney Transplant
Discover new possibilities for health and living

CHAPTER 1

YOUR JOURNEY WITH LUPUS NEPHRITIS

YOU ARE NOT ALONE—STRENGTH AND HOPE ARE ALWAYS WITHIN REACH

Abstract

Lupus Nephritis is not just a diagnosis—it is a profound life shift that touches every part of a patient's world. This guide was written to offer more than medical facts; it extends a hand of hope to patients, families, and caregivers navigating this journey. Through clear guidance and, Leah's powerful story of resilience, it reminds readers that strength is found in the darkest moments. With the support of family, faith, and compassionate care, life with Lupus Nephritis can be faced with courage, not fear. You are not alone. Like Leah's, your story is still being written—with hope at every turn.

Keywords: Lupus nephritis, hope, resilience, patient empowerment

Lupus Nephritis is a chronic illness. It affects approximately one million people worldwide. Approximately 50% of patients with Lupus will develop Lupus Nephritis in their lifetime. Lupus Nephritis presents several difficulties and alters the way of life. This chronic demanding condition affects the patients and their loved ones. The caregivers of those affected by this disease also face the challenges that come with it. This book aims to be more than just a source of information. Patients, relatives, and caregivers will find it a helpful companion as they navigate the challenges of lupus nephritis. We aim to provide you with the knowledge, skills, and support you need to understand your condition and thrive despite its challenges.

Purpose of the Guide and What Patients, Families, and Caregivers Can Learn

Lupus nephritis is a complex disease. There are moments when the medical jargon, available treatments, and regular doctor visits seem overwhelming. By offering simple, understandable, and accessible explanations, this book seeks to close the knowledge gap between patients and the illness. By educating you, we hope to enable you to take control of your health. This guide will help you navigate your everyday life with Lupus Nephritis, from receiving the diagnosis of Lupus Nephritis, navigating the treatment options, making the most out of the doctor visits, and finding ways to live your best life with this chronic condition.

This book is a valuable resource for patients, answering commonly asked concerns and outlining treatment options, lifestyle changes, and the importance of actively participating in your care plan. It seeks to simplify the condition and help you comprehend your doctor's advice. We encourage you to discuss any changes you wish to consider with your doctors. You'll also find helpful tips for managing your medications, recognizing early warning signs of complications, and maintaining a healthy lifestyle to support your treatment.

This book offers families and caregivers great insights on how to effectively help their loved ones as they battle with this complicated disease. It underlines the emotional impact Lupus Nephritis may have on individuals. It provides proactive ways for caregivers to assist them in managing the disease's physical and emotional challenges. We understand that caring for someone with a chronic illness can sometimes feel daunting. The most effective strategy to fight burnout is to know the condition better and help your loved ones navigate this complicated lifelong path. This book will provide perspective from a young patient diagnosed with Lupus Nephritis and her journey with this disease and living her life with this new condition.

Introduction to Lupus Nephritis and Its Impact on Daily Life

Lupus Nephritis is a condition that affects the kidneys in people with systemic lupus erythematosus, also called lupus, an autoimmune disease. In autoimmune conditions like lupus, the immune system, which usually defends the body against infections, mistakenly attacks its own body tissues. In the case of Lupus Nephritis, this attack is directed at the kidneys, leading to inflammation and, if left untreated, causing damage to the kidney and kidney failure.

The kidneys filter waste from the blood and maintain the body's balance of fluids and electrolytes. Lupus Nephritis disrupts this process, which can lead to a range of health issues. For some individuals, the progression of the disease is slow, with minimal symptoms at first. However, in other cases, the disease can worsen rapidly, leading to chronic kidney disease or even end-stage kidney disease, i.e., kidney failure, a situation that may require treatments such as dialysis or a kidney transplant.

Lupus Nephritis can significantly impact daily life. Fatigue is one of the most common symptoms, making even simple activities difficult to manage. The unpredictability of the disease, with flare-ups that can occur without warning, adds a layer of emotional stress. This unpredictability can affect a person’s social life, work, and family responsibilities, making it harder to plan or feel in control. During flare-ups, individuals may experience increased anxiety, frustration, or a sense of emotional exhaustion.

Many people with Lupus Nephritis face not only the physical challenges of the disease but also the emotional and psychological hurdles that come with managing a long-term illness. It’s common for individuals to feel isolated, anxious, or even depressed, especially as they adjust to life with a chronic disease. This book also addresses these emotional aspects and offers guidance on coping with the challenges and finding a balance that supports physical and mental well-being while living with Lupus Nephritis.

Leah's Story: A Journey of Courage, Family, and Hope

Leah was a vibrant freshman, a young woman whose life was stitched together with music, laughter, and simple joys. Her future felt bright, filled with dreams yet to be realized.

The first hints of trouble were quiet and easy to dismiss — stomach discomfort, skin breakouts—minor inconveniences, nothing more. But then, during a family vacation in June, just as the world was slowly emerging from the first brutal wave of COVID-19, Leah’s body betrayed her. Crippling joint pains seized her limbs. Ice brought no relief. Her strength drained away overnight. She was bedridden, helpless, and terrified.

Within weeks, Leah’s health spiraled. Blood tests revealed liver enzymes had doubled. High fevers, yellowing eyes, nausea, relentless vomiting, and weight loss consumed her summer. Her urine turned dark and foamy. Her skin itched uncontrollably. Even the simple act of speaking left her trembling with exhaustion. Once a bright, energetic soul, Leah was now imprisoned in a body that seemed to be crumbling from within.

Urgent care visits, ER trips, primary care appointments — each offered hope, and each ended with more confusion. Diagnoses ranged from viral infections to tick-borne illnesses. She endured countless blood draws and tests, but answers remained elusive. By August, she could barely move without pain, and sleep became a distant memory.

A terrifying ER visit led to Leah's first hospital admission. Invasive tests followed — including a bone marrow biopsy to rule out leukemia. She hallucinated from fever and medication, lost in confusion and fear. Transferred in an ambulance, strapped down and unable to move, she felt more alone than ever.

At a tertiary hospital, after months of searching, doctors finally uncovered the truth: Leah had stage IV lupus nephritis. Her immune system was attacking her kidneys with ruthless efficiency. The diagnosis felt overwhelming — a mixture of relief to have answers and fear of what lay ahead.

Hospitalization during COVID was its agony. Leah lay isolated for months, her only visitors the masked faces of nurses and doctors. No parents. No siblings. No familiar touch. Only the compassion of a few remarkable nurses broke through the loneliness — a nurse who sneaked her a meal she craved, a hand on her shoulder when words were not enough.

Through it all, Leah's family became her unseen anchor. Though they couldn't be physically present, their love filled the hospital walls. Daily phone calls, whispered prayers, messages of unwavering hope — they fought for her spirit when her body was too weak to fight for itself.

Her mother, especially, became her guardian angel — ready to care for Leah day and night once she returned home. Her siblings, her friends, her church community: they never let her forget that she was still loved, still whole, still Leah.

Her healthcare team, too, was extraordinary. They treated her not just with medication but with humanity. They took time to explain complex medical terms, to listen to her fears, to hold space for her grief. Their compassion gave Leah the courage to step into the unknown to believe that healing was possible.

Treatment was grueling — five days of high-dose steroids, a slow taper, and immunosuppressants like Cellcept and Plaquenil. Her skin became painfully sensitive. Her hair fell out in clumps. Her muscles were wasted to the point that even sitting upright felt like climbing a mountain. Wheelchairs, shower chairs, sleepless nights — these became her new normal.

Returning home was not a triumphant ending but the beginning of a new battle. Leah's mother slept beside her each night, monitoring her breathing and calming her racing heart during panic attacks. Daily blood pressure checks triggered waves of anxiety. Chest pains blurred the line between fear and reality. For a long time, even the idea of returning to her "normal life" felt like a distant dream.

Depression settled in, especially during the long, dark winters. Leah hated what Lupus had stolen from her. She grieved her independence, her hair, and her plans.

She feared becoming "the girl with lupus," defined only by her disease.

But slowly, painfully, Leah rebuilt her life. She learned to listen to her body. She allowed herself to rest. She reconnected with friends, even if only by text. She taught herself to accept help without shame. And most importantly, she remembered that lupus might shape her life — but it would never define her.

Today, Leah is still healing. Her kidney function remains stable. Her days are again filled with music lessons, movie nights, and quiet hope. She cherishes simple moments, knowing now how precious they are. Her faith, her family, and the extraordinary kindness of her healthcare team carried her through the darkest valleys.

Leah's story is not just about surviving a devastating illness. It is a story of transformation — a testimony to the healing power of love, community, faith, and resilience.

It reminds every patient reading this book: You are not alone. You are not your diagnosis.

Like Leah, your story is still unfolding — filled with chapters of courage, chapters of hope, and chapters still unwritten.

Key Statistics and Facts about Lupus Nephritis

Leah's journey is truly personal, but it also tells a bigger story that resonates with many individuals with lupus nephritis. Although each person's experience is distinct, the hurdles she encountered — from her diagnosis to her emotional healing — reflect the realities faced by millions around the globe. To grasp the full scope and significance of lupus nephritis, it's essential to consider the wider facts, trends, and outcomes that impact the lives of patients and their families daily.

Lupus Nephritis is a severe form of systemic lupus erythematosus. It's estimated that 40-60% of those with lupus will experience some type of Lupus Nephritis at some point in their lives, highlighting the significant impact that Lupus Nephritis has on lupus patients globally (1, 2). Lupus Nephritis happens when the immune system mistakenly targets the kidneys, leading to inflammation and kidney damage. If not appropriately treated, Lupus Nephritis may progress to chronic kidney disease or even kidney failure, which might require dialysis or a kidney transplant (3). Studies show that 10-30% of patients with lupus nephritis will progress to kidney failure, requiring dialysis or a kidney transplant (4, 5). The effects of kidney failure from lupus nephritis are especially significant since 3/4th of those affected are under the age of 50 (6). The risk of kidney failure in lupus nephritis improved from the 1970s to the mid-1990s, followed by a period of stability and a rise in the late 2000s. This trend indicates there may be challenges in the effectiveness or accessibility of current treatments (3). However, there have been multiple new medications approved for the treatment of Lupus Nephritis in the past 3 years, which should lead to decreasing the risk of kidney failure in patients with Lupus Nephritis

The disease is disproportionately prevalent among women, particularly those from African American, Hispanic, Asian, and Native American backgrounds. Studies have shown that African American women with lupus are at significantly higher risk of developing Lupus Nephritis compared to other racial or ethnic groups (7, 8). This group also tends to present with more severe forms of the disease and experiences worse outcomes, including a higher likelihood of developing kidney failure (8).

Lupus primarily impacts women during their reproductive years. 2/3rd of patients with lupus start experiencing symptoms between the ages of 16 and 55. Twenty percent of people experience symptoms before turning 16, while 15 percent experience symptoms appear after age 55 (9, 10).

Conclusion

In conclusion, while Lupus Nephritis can present its challenges, it's important to remember that it doesn't define someone. The journey might sometimes feel daunting, but with the correct information, support, treatment plan, and medical team, you can manage Lupus Nephritis and enjoy a fulfilling life. This guide offers clear and practical insights to help you, and your loved ones make informed choices, understand medical terminology, and navigate the complexities of diagnosis, treatment, and lifestyle adjustments. You can keep the disease from taking over your life with an appropriate treatment plan, regular check-ups, and a proactive approach to managing symptoms. Knowledge is empowering, and with the resources in this book, you'll be well-prepared to take charge of your health and well-being.

Lupus Nephritis diagnosis can be life changing. It is essential to remember that people with lupus nephritis survive and live a fulfilling life everyone deserves. The emotional and physical hurdles may seem overwhelming, but having resilience and a strong support network can make a difference. Whether through family, friends, support groups, or healthcare professionals, seeking help is a sign of strength. Understanding that you are not alone on this journey is vital. Others with Lupus Nephritis have walked similar paths, and their stories remind us of the incredible strength of the human spirit. You can lead a fulfilling life despite the challenges by adapting to new realities, embracing the journey with patience and determination, and taking control of your treatment plan. Trust the process, celebrate the small wins along the way, and remember that every step, no matter how tiny, brings you closer to a healthier, happier future.

References

1. Hoover PJ, Costenbader KH. Insights into the epidemiology and management of lupus nephritis from the US rheumatologist's perspective. Kidney Int. 2016;90(3):487-92.
2. Ward MM. Prevalence of physician-diagnosed systemic lupus erythematosus in the United States: results from the third national health and nutrition examination survey. J Womens Health (Larchmt). 2004;13(6):713-8.
3. Tektonidou MG, Dasgupta A, Ward MM. Risk of Endstage Renal Disease in Patients With Lupus Nephritis, 1971-2015: A Systematic

Review and Bayesian Meta-Analysis. Arthritis Rheumatol. 2016;68(6):1432-41.
4. Lateef A, Petri M. Unmet medical needs in systemic lupus erythematosus. Arthritis Res Ther. 2012;14 Suppl 4(Suppl 4):S4.
5. Croca SC, Rodrigues T, Isenberg DA. Assessment of a lupus nephritis cohort over a 30-year period. Rheumatology (Oxford). 2011;50(8):1424-30.
6. Ward MM. Medical insurance, socioeconomic status, and age of onset of endstage renal disease in patients with lupus nephritis. J Rheumatol. 2007;34(10):2024-7.
7. Parikh SV, Almaani S, Brodsky S, Rovin BH. Update on Lupus Nephritis: Core Curriculum 2020. Am J Kidney Dis. 2020;76(2): 265-81.
8. Contreras G, Lenz O, Pardo V, Borja E, Cely C, Iqbal K, et al. Outcomes in African Americans and Hispanics with lupus nephritis. Kidney Int. 2006;69(10):1846-51.
9. Ballou SP, Khan MA, Kushner I. Clinical features of systemic lupus erythematosus: differences related to race and age of onset. Arthritis Rheum. 1982;25(1):55-60.
10. Maningding E, Dall'Era M, Trupin L, Murphy LB, Yazdany J. Racial and Ethnic Differences in the Prevalence and Time to Onset of Manifestations of Systemic Lupus Erythematosus: The California Lupus Surveillance Project. Arthritis Care Res (Hoboken). 2020;72(5):622-9.

CHAPTER 2

WHEN LUPUS AFFECTS THE KIDNEYS

UNDERSTAND HOW LUPUS CHANGES KIDNEY HEALTH

Abstract

This chapter introduces readers to the fundamentals of lupus nephritis by weaving together a story and clear scientific explanation. It describes how systemic lupus erythematosus (SLE) affects the immune system and can lead to widespread organ damage, particularly the kidneys. The chapter highlights the importance of early detection and monitoring of kidney involvement in lupus patients, discusses the autoimmune mechanisms behind lupus nephritis, and compares it to other kidney diseases. Blending storytelling with medical facts empowers patients to recognize symptoms early and underscores the critical need for proactive management to prevent long-term kidney damage.

Keywords: systemic lupus erythematosus, Autoimmunity, Kidney inflammation, early detection, patient empowerment, proactive care

It was 3:00 AM when Leah, a bright freshman student full of dreams and plans, awoke drenched in sweat. Her body ached as if it had been battered from the inside out, and catching her breath felt like trying to breathe through thick fog. A sharp, throbbing discomfort stabbed at her lower back, and when she tried to swing her legs out of bed, she gasped — her ankles were grotesquely swollen, almost unrecognizable as if they were filled with heavy sand.

Over the past few months, Leah had been grappling with scattered symptoms — aching joints, stubborn fatigue, occasional swelling — but she had brushed them aside. She was young. Busy. Life was supposed to be moving forward, not slipping from under her.

But tonight felt different. Darker. More urgent. Something deep within her told her that whatever was happening wouldn't be fixed by a few days of rest or a bottle of over-the-counter medicine.

Leah stumbled to the bathroom, her legs trembling. A glance in the mirror stole her breath. Her face was puffy, and her eyes were barely recognizable under the swelling. The faint butterfly-shaped rash across her cheeks, blazing like a warning signal she could no longer ignore. As she leaned closer, she noticed something else — her urine, darker than ever, almost tea-colored, and far less in volume than it should have been.

Then came a sudden, crushing ache in her chest, and for a terrifying moment, Leah clutched the sink for support. A frightening thought whispered into her mind — *could her kidneys be failing?*

But Leah had no name for what was happening inside her. She didn't know yet that her immune system, designed to protect her, had turned into her greatest enemy. She didn't know she was living with lupus — and that now, lupus had found its way to her kidneys.

The next few weeks became a blur of urgent care visits, emergency rooms, endless blood draws, and specialist consultations. Each time, the doctors were kind but puzzled. They ran tests and prescribed medications for symptoms, but no one could explain why Leah's body seemed to be falling apart piece by piece.

With every unanswered question, Leah's fear grew. She knew, deep down, that time was running out. Without a diagnosis, without a clear direction, she could lose her kidneys — or worse.

For so many patients, lupus does not arrive with a grand announcement. It creeps in slowly, subtly — a swollen ankle here, a rash there, a fatigue so deep it feels like drowning — until a tipping point is reached. By the time the signs are unmistakable, critical damage may already be underway.

Without early detection and aggressive management, lupus nephritis — the kidney inflammation caused by lupus — can silently destroy kidney function, leading to kidney failure, dialysis, or even the need for a transplant. It's a harsh betrayal: the body's immune defenses turning inward, attacking the very organs meant to sustain life.

Finally, after one particularly alarming hospitalization, Leah's life changed. She was transferred to a tertiary care hospital, where a team of specialists — including rheumatologists and nephrologists — worked together to solve the puzzle. Blood tests, kidney biopsies, and careful evaluations led to a name for her suffering: Systemic Lupus Erythematosus, with active lupus nephritis already damaging her kidneys.

The diagnosis was overwhelming, but it was also a lifeline. For Leah, having a name for her enemy meant a plan could be made. It meant there was hope.

This chapter will explore these conditions in greater detail, offering knowledge, hope, and a path forward for all who face this journey.

Introduction to Systemic Lupus Erythematosus as a Chronic Autoimmune Disease

Systemic Lupus Erythematosus, or in simple words, lupus, is a chronic autoimmune condition where the immune system mistakenly attacks the body's tissues. The immune system protects against infections and harmful invaders like bacteria and viruses, but in people with lupus, the immune system confuses healthy body tissues for threats. This misidentification produces autoantibodies—proteins that harm healthy cells instead of targeting invaders. Consequently, this self-attack causes widespread inflammation and damage to various organs, so lupus is considered a multisystemic disease (affecting multiple organs).

One of the challenges of lupus is the unpredictable nature of this disease. The disease usually goes through cycles of flares—times when symptoms worsen—followed by remissions when symptoms lessen or even disappear. It's often hard to identify the causes of these flares, but stress, infections, sun exposure, or hormonal changes can trigger them. This unpredictability makes managing lupus a bit more challenging, as patients must continually adjust to changing symptoms and levels of disease activity.

How Lupus Affects Multiple Organs and Systems in the Body

Lupus is a systemic disease since it has the potential to impact almost every organ in the body. The extent and combination of affected systems can differ significantly from one individual to another, which means that each person with lupus is unique. Some individuals might experience mild symptoms involving just one organ system, while others could have serious, life-threatening complications (1-3). Here’s a closer look at how lupus can influence various body parts (table 1).

Table 1: Effect of Lupus on body systems

Organ/System	Effect of Lupus
Skin	• Commonly affected by rashes (e.g., malar or butterfly rash across cheeks and nose) • Photosensitivity worsens with sun exposure • Discoid rashes (thick, scaly patches) • Possible hair loss during flare-ups
Joints	• Joint pain and inflammation (arthralgia, arthritis) • Symmetrical pain in small joints (e.g., hands, wrists, knees) • Morning stiffness • Limited mobility, affecting daily tasks
Heart	• Inflammation around the heart (pericarditis) causing chest pain • Myocarditis (inflammation of the heart muscle) • Increased risk of atherosclerosis (leading to heart attacks and strokes)
Lungs	• Pleuritis (inflammation of lung membranes) causing chest pain • Lupus pneumonitis with fever, cough, and difficulty breathing • Pulmonary hypertension (increased pressure in arteries in the lungs) and interstitial lung disease in severe cases
Kidneys	• Lupus nephritis (inflammation in kidneys)
Blood	• Anemia (leading to fatigue and weakness) • Thrombocytopenia (low platelet count), causing easy bruising • Leukopenia (low white blood cell count), increasing infection risk • Blood clots
Nervous system	• Neuropsychiatric lupus causes headaches, seizures, confusion, and memory issues • Severe cases may involve lupus cerebritis (brain inflammation) • Peripheral neuropathy (numbness/tingling in extremities)

1. Skin:

The skin is one of the organs most frequently impacted by lupus. Cutaneous or skin lupus describes how lupus appears on the skin. Many individuals with lupus experience skin rashes, which can worsen with sun exposure—a sensitivity known as photosensitivity. Lupus's most recognizable skin symptom is the malar rash, which spreads across the cheeks and nose, often called the butterfly rash. While this rash is distinctive and usually painless, it can be a visible sign of the disease's activity.

Along with the malar rash, patients might notice other skin issues like discoid rashes—these are thick, scaly patches that can show up, especially on areas that get a lot of sun, such as the face, neck, and arms. Some people may also face hair loss, which can be temporary during flare-ups or more lasting if lupus-related inflammation affects the scalp.

Photosensitivity can make it challenging to enjoy outdoor activities, as even a little sun exposure might trigger flare-ups. That's why it's often recommended for those with lupus to use sunscreen, wear protective clothing, and limit time in direct sunlight.

2. Joints:

Joint pain and inflammation, commonly known as arthralgia or arthritis, are frequently seen in lupus and can be some of the first signs. This pain usually impacts several joints and is often symmetrical, affecting the same joints on both sides. The small joints in the hands, wrists, and knees are the most common, but other joints can also be affected.

Although lupus-related arthritis may lead to swelling, stiffness, and reduced mobility, it typically doesn't result in the same level of joint damage found in other autoimmune disorders, such as rheumatoid arthritis. Nonetheless, joint pain can still significantly affect a person's capacity to carry out everyday activities. Simple tasks like holding a pen, typing, or opening a jar can become challenging during a flare.

Morning stiffness is a common symptom of joint inflammation associated with lupus. Many patients report waking up with stiff, painful joints that gradually loosen as the day progresses. This stiffness can disrupt work and everyday activities, making joint pain one of the most challenging aspects of living with the disease for numerous individuals.

3. Heart:

Lupus can lead to inflammation in and around the heart, a condition called pericarditis (the inflammation of the sac surrounding the heart). This can result in sharp chest pain, mainly when lying down or taking a deep breath, and may also cause shortness of breath. In certain situations, fluid might build up around the heart, known as pericardial effusion, and it can be severe if not addressed quickly.

Lupus can also lead to myocarditis (inflammation of the heart muscle) and endocarditis (inflammation of the heart's inner lining), affecting how well the heart functions. As time goes on, lupus may increase the risk of atherosclerosis (narrowing of the arteries due to plaque buildup), which heightens the chances of heart attacks and strokes (4, 5). Research indicates that people with lupus face a much greater risk of developing cardiovascular disease compared to the general population, so taking care of heart health is crucial in managing lupus (4, 6).

4. Lungs:

Lupus often impacts the lungs and the surrounding membrane, leading to issues like pleuritis (inflammation of the pleura) and lupus pneumonitis (inflammation within the lung tissue). Pleuritis can cause sharp chest pain that worsens with deep breaths or coughing, while lupus pneumonitis might bring on fever, coughing, and trouble breathing.

In more severe situations, lupus can result in pulmonary hypertension (high blood pressure in the lung arteries) or interstitial lung disease, hindering oxygen exchange and making breathing more challenging over time. Ongoing lung involvement in lupus can significantly affect a person's quality of life and, if not addressed, may lead to severe complications (7-10).

5. Kidneys:

The kidneys are among the most vulnerable organs in patients with lupus. Approximately half of the people with lupus will develop Lupus Nephritis, a serious condition in which the kidneys become inflamed due to the immune system's attack on kidney tissue. The kidneys are responsible for filtering waste and excess fluids from the blood, and when they are damaged, this critical function becomes impaired. Because Lupus Nephritis is a common and serious manifestation of lupus, regular monitoring of kidney function through urine and blood tests is essential for all lupus patients (11, 12).

6. Blood and Blood Vessels:

Lupus can impact the blood and blood vessels in various ways. Many people with lupus experience anemia, a condition without healthy red blood cells to deliver sufficient oxygen to the body's tissues, often resulting in fatigue and weakness. Furthermore, lupus can lead to thrombocytopenia (a low platelet count), which might cause easy bruising, nosebleeds, or longer bleeding from cuts.

Patients with lupus might experience leukopenia (a low white blood cell count), which can increase their vulnerability to infections. A significant complication of lupus is the formation of blood clots, especially in those with antiphospholipid antibodies. This condition, referred to as antiphospholipid syndrome, heightens the risk of blood clots in the legs (deep vein thrombosis), lungs (pulmonary embolism), and brain (stroke).

7. Nervous System:

Lupus can also impact the central nervous system (CNS) and peripheral nervous system (PNS), leading to neurological symptoms. Neuropsychiatric lupus refers to the involvement of the nervous system in lupus, which can cause symptoms such as headaches, seizures, confusion, memory problems, and mood swings.

Some patients may experience more severe neurological complications, such as lupus cerebritis, which can cause inflammation in the brain and lead to cognitive dysfunction. In contrast, others may develop peripheral neuropathy, causing numbness or tingling in the hands and feet (13, 14).

Common Symptoms of Lupus

Lupus presents with a wide array of symptoms that can vary significantly from one person to another. Some of the most common symptoms include (3):

- **Joint pain and stiffness**, particularly in the hands, wrists, and knees.
- **Fatigue** that can be debilitating is often described as a deep, unrelenting tiredness.
- **Skin rashes**, including the malar (butterfly) rash, may worsen with sun exposure.

- **Hair loss** can range from mild thinning to more noticeable bald patches.
- **Fever**, often without an apparent infection, indicates disease activity.
- **Swelling in the legs or around the eyes** may be an early sign of kidney involvement.
- **Cognitive issues**, or "lupus fog," affect memory and concentration.

These symptoms, among others, highlight how unique lupus is for each person, which means that a personalized treatment plan is necessary for everyone. Both patients and healthcare providers need to grasp the complex nature of lupus to create effective management strategies.

Connection of Lupus-to-Lupus Nephritis

As discussed earlier, one of the most significant and potentially life-threatening complications of lupus is the development of Lupus Nephritis, which specifically impacts the kidneys. Lupus Nephritis occurs when the immune system's abnormal attack on the body targets the kidneys, leading to inflammation, tissue damage, and impaired kidney function. This condition is one of lupus's most common organ-specific manifestations and occurs in 40-60% of individuals diagnosed with lupus (15, 16).

For numerous patients, the beginning of Lupus Nephritis can be subtle and gradual. Some individuals might notice symptoms early on, while others may not show any clear signs of kidney issues for years, highlighting the importance of regular check-ups. If not diagnosed and treated in time, Lupus Nephritis can lead to permanent kidney damage, resulting in chronic kidney disease or even end-stage renal disease, which could require dialysis or a kidney transplant.

It is essential for patients, their families, and healthcare professionals to recognize the link between lupus and Lupus Nephritis. The kidneys play a crucial role in filtering waste from the blood and keeping fluids and electrolytes balanced, so any issues with their function can significantly impact overall health. In lupus, the immune system's assault on the kidneys leads to inflammation in the glomeruli, the kidney's filtering units. This can cause damage that worsens over time if not effectively managed.

Importance of Early Detection and Monitoring of Kidney Involvement in Lupus Patients

One of the essential aspects of managing lupus is the early detection and ongoing monitoring of kidney involvement, as early Lupus Nephritis can often be quite subtle. The kidneys can become inflamed without presenting any apparent symptoms, especially in the early stages, which means patients might not realize there are kidney issues until significant damage has occurred. That's why individuals with lupus must undergo regular kidney function tests as part of their routine healthcare.

Early detection allows healthcare providers to intervene promptly, initiating treatments that can reduce inflammation and prevent further damage. Without early detection, Lupus Nephritis can progress to more severe forms, where the risk of permanent kidney damage becomes significantly higher. Delayed diagnosis can also lead to complications such as fluid retention, high blood pressure, and accumulation of toxins in the blood, all of which can affect other organs in the body and reduce the patient's quality of life. We'll discuss the tests used to identify involvement in the upcoming chapters.

Breakdown of How the Immune System Affects the Kidneys

Normal Immune System Function:

The immune system is like the body's superhero squad, always on the lookout to shield us from harmful invaders such as bacteria, viruses, fungi, and toxins. A healthy person works smoothly, identifying these unwelcome guests through a sophisticated network of immune cells and proteins that collaborate to spot, neutralize, and remove threats. When pathogens try to invade, the immune system sends in its specialized troops, like white blood cells (leukocytes), which include T-cells, B-cells, and macrophages, to tackle the danger.

A vital part of our defense system involves the creation of antibodies, which are special proteins made by B-cells. These antibodies are crafted to attach to antigens—molecules found on the surface of foreign invaders—and signal them for elimination. When the antigen-antibody complex forms, it triggers a response from the immune system, destroying the invader through the teamwork of immune cells and complement proteins that enhance the immune response. What's impressive is that the immune system can distinguish between self (the body's tissues) and non-self (foreign invaders), enabling it to target harmful intruders while keeping our cells safe.

However, autoimmune diseases such as systemic lupus erythematosus (SLE) lose this critical distinction between self and non-self. The immune system begins to malfunction, resulting in a misguided attack on the body's healthy tissues. In the case of Lupus Nephritis, this attack is directed explicitly at the kidneys, leading to inflammation and progressive damage.

Autoimmune Response in Lupus Nephritis:

In individuals with lupus, the immune system becomes overactive and mistakenly targets healthy tissues, including vital organs such as the kidneys. The underlying mechanism of this immune dysfunction involves the production of autoantibodies—antibodies that target the body's cells and tissues rather than foreign invaders. These autoantibodies play a central role in developing Lupus Nephritis, as they initiate the inflammatory process that damages the kidneys.

Two specific autoantibodies are particularly relevant to Lupus Nephritis:

1. **Antinuclear antibodies (ANA)**: These are a broad class of autoantibodies that target proteins inside the nucleus of the body's cells. ANAs are present in nearly all individuals with lupus, making them a key marker for the disease, although they are not specific to Lupus Nephritis alone. ANAs attack various tissues throughout the body, leading to the systemic nature of lupus, which can affect multiple organs.
2. **Anti-double-stranded DNA (anti-dsDNA) antibodies**: These autoantibodies target the body's DNA, particularly the double-stranded DNA found within cells. Anti-dsDNA antibodies are particular to lupus and are directly implicated in developing Lupus Nephritis. High levels of anti-dsDNA antibodies are often associated with increased disease activity and kidney involvement. These antibodies form immune complexes by binding to DNA fragments released by dying cells.

Formation and Deposition of Immune Complexes in the Kidneys:

The process by which immune complexes form and deposit in the kidneys is at the heart of Lupus Nephritis. When autoantibodies like anti-dsDNA antibodies circulate in the bloodstream, they bind to DNA or other nuclear material released by damaged or dying cells. These antigen-antibody complexes are immune complexes, and their formation is a hallmark of many autoimmune diseases, including lupus.

Once these immune complexes are formed, they circulate in the blood. They can become deposited in the glomeruli—the tiny filtering units in the kidneys that are responsible for filtering blood to remove waste, excess fluids, and electrolytes. The glomeruli are composed of a network of tiny blood vessels that allow the passage of blood while retaining essential proteins and nutrients. In Lupus Nephritis, however, these immune complexes accumulate in the glomeruli, triggering a localized immune response that leads to inflammation and damage.

The immune system sends white blood cells, such as macrophages and T-cells, to the deposition site to eliminate these immune complexes. These immune cells release inflammatory cytokines and other signaling molecules, further escalating the inflammatory response. As this inflammation persists, it causes the glomerular membranes to become thickened and damaged, compromising their ability to perform their essential filtering function.

Kidney Inflammation and Damage:

The inflammation caused by the deposition of immune complexes in the kidneys directly damages the glomeruli and other parts of the kidneys. This inflammation, known as glomerulonephritis, is characterized by swelling, increased permeability of the glomerular membranes, and the activation of additional immune cells that perpetuate the damage.

Over time, the continuous inflammatory process leads to structural damage in the kidneys, impairing their ability to filter blood properly. The damaged glomeruli allow substances that are typically retained in the bloodstream—such as proteins and red blood cells—to leak into the urine, resulting in the following common symptoms of Lupus Nephritis:

1. **Proteinuria (Protein in the Urine)**: Proteinuria is among the earliest and most common signs of Lupus Nephritis. Under normal circumstances, the kidneys prevent large proteins, such as albumin, from filtering into the urine. However, when the glomerular membranes are damaged by inflammation, they become more permeable, allowing proteins to pass through and be excreted in the urine. This leads to foamy or bubbly urine, a visible sign of proteinuria.

Over time, significant protein loss can lead to nephrotic syndrome, characterized by extreme protein loss, swelling (edema) in the legs and around the eyes, low blood protein levels, and increased cholesterol levels.

2. **Hematuria (Blood in the Urine)**: Hematuria, or blood in the urine, occurs when the kidney's inflammation causes red blood cells to leak into the urine. This may result in urine that appears pink, red, or cola-colored. Hematuria can be a sign of significant damage to the glomeruli and is another important indicator of kidney involvement in Lupus Nephritis.
   In some cases, hematuria may not be visible to the naked eye but can be detected through microscopic urine examination.
3. **Reduced Kidney Function**: As the inflammation progresses and more damage is inflicted on the kidneys, their ability to filter waste products from the blood becomes impaired. This leads to a buildup of waste in the blood, which can cause fatigue, nausea, and other symptoms of kidney dysfunction. In more severe cases, the persistent inflammation and resulting tissue damage can lead to scarring of the kidneys, a condition known as glomerulosclerosis.

If left untreated, Lupus Nephritis can progress to chronic kidney disease, which is characterized by a gradual decline in kidney function over time. In the advanced stages, CKD can progress to end-stage kidney disease, where the kidneys lose nearly all their filtering capacity, requiring patients to undergo dialysis or a kidney transplant to maintain their health.

How Lupus Nephritis Differs from Other Kidney Diseases

Lupus Nephritis is a unique and complex form of kidney disease that arises precisely from the autoimmune condition lupus. While many other kidney diseases may affect kidney function, Lupus Nephritis stands apart due to its autoimmune origin, the systemic nature of lupus, and its fluctuating course of disease activity. Understanding the distinctions between Lupus Nephritis and other autoimmune and non—autoimmune kidney diseases is essential for proper diagnosis, treatment, and management.

Comparison with Other Autoimmune Kidney Diseases:

1. IgA Nephropathy: IgA nephropathy, also known as Berger's disease, is another autoimmune condition that affects the kidneys, but there are significant differences between it and Lupus Nephritis.

Immune Complex Deposits: In IgA nephropathy, the immune complexes that deposit in the kidneys consist of IgA antibodies produced in response to infections or environmental triggers. These immune complexes accumulate in the mesangium (supportive tissue inside the tiny filtering units of the kidneys), leading to inflammation and damage. In contrast, Lupus Nephritis involves the deposition of antinuclear antibodies (ANA) and anti-dsDNA antibodies in the glomeruli (the filtering part of the kidney), where they trigger an inflammatory response.

Systemic Involvement: One of the critical differences between IgA nephropathy and Lupus Nephritis is that IgA nephropathy is primarily a localized kidney disease. At the same time, Lupus Nephritis is part of the lupus. Patients with Lupus Nephritis often experience symptoms that affect other organs, such as the skin, joints, heart, and lungs, making it a multi-organ disease. IgA nephropathy, on the other hand, typically only affects the kidneys and does not have widespread systemic effects.

2. Anti GBM disease (Goodpasture syndrome): Anti GBM disease, another autoimmune disease, primarily affects both the kidneys and the lungs, but it presents differently from Lupus Nephritis.

Autoantibody Targets: In anti GBM disease, the immune system produces autoantibodies that specifically target the glomerular basement membrane (The glomerular basement membrane is a thin, protective layer in the kidneys' tiny filtering units) in the kidneys and the alveolar basement membrane) The alveolar basement membrane is a thin layer found in the lungs, specifically in the small air sacs called alveoli) in the lungs. These autoantibodies are known as anti-glomerular basement membrane (anti-GBM) antibodies, and their attack results in severe kidney damage and bleeding into the lungs (pulmonary hemorrhage). In Lupus Nephritis, however, the immune system targets various nuclear components through anti-dsDNA antibodies and other autoantibodies, and the immune complex deposits are not restricted to the glomerular basement membrane.

Systemic Nature: Anti GBM disease is less systemic than Lupus Nephritis. While anti GBM disease affects both the kidneys and the lungs, Lupus Nephritis is part of lupus's broader systemic disease process, which can affect multiple organs beyond the kidneys and lungs, including the heart, skin, joints, and nervous system.

Presentation: Anti GBM disease often presents with rapidly progressive glomerulonephritis, leading to a fast decline in kidney function, whereas

Lupus Nephritis can follow a more variable course, with episodes of flares and remissions.

Non-Autoimmune Kidney Diseases:

1. Diabetic Nephropathy: Diabetic nephropathy is one of the most common causes of chronic kidney disease worldwide, particularly in patients with long-standing diabetes mellitus. However, the mechanisms driving diabetic nephropathy differ substantially from those in Lupus Nephritis.

Etiology: Diabetic nephropathy is caused by chronic hyperglycemia (high blood sugar), which leads to structural and functional changes in the kidneys, such as thickening of the glomerular basement membrane, expansion of the mesangial matrix, and sclerosis of the glomeruli. In Lupus Nephritis, kidney damage is driven by an immune-mediated attack rather than metabolic factors.

Progression: Diabetic nephropathy typically follows a slow, progressive decline in kidney function over many years, with persistent proteinuria as an early sign. Lupus Nephritis, on the other hand, can fluctuate, with periods of rapid deterioration (flares) followed by stabilization or remission.

Systemic Involvement: Diabetic nephropathy primarily affects the kidneys, although patients with diabetes can develop complications in other organs (e.g., heart, eyes, nerves). Lupus Nephritis, part of a systemic autoimmune disease, often involves multiple organ systems beyond the kidneys.

2. Hypertensive Nephrosclerosis: Hypertensive nephrosclerosis refers to kidney damage caused by chronic high blood pressure. While both hypertensive nephrosclerosis and Lupus Nephritis lead to kidney dysfunction, the underlying causes and disease mechanisms are quite different.

Etiology: In hypertensive nephrosclerosis, the high pressure in the blood vessels supplying the kidneys causes damage to the small arteries and arterioles, leading to ischemia (reduced blood flow) and scarring in the kidney tissue. This is a mechanical process driven by pressure, unlike the immune-mediated inflammation seen in Lupus Nephritis.

Progression: Hypertensive nephrosclerosis tends to progress gradually because of long-term, uncontrolled high blood pressure. In contrast, Lupus

Nephritis may progress more unpredictably, with flares of acute kidney inflammation followed by periods of relative inactivity.

Treatment Focus: The treatment of hypertensive nephrosclerosis revolves around blood pressure control to prevent further kidney damage. While blood pressure control is also essential in Lupus Nephritis, the primary treatment involves immunosuppressive therapy to reduce the autoimmune response that drives kidney inflammation.

Unique Features of Lupus Nephritis:

1. Multi-Organ Involvement: One of the defining characteristics of Lupus Nephritis is that it occurs as part of the broader systemic disease lupus. Unlike many other kidney diseases limited to the kidneys, Lupus Nephritis is just one manifestation of a disease that can affect multiple organ systems.

Complexity in Treatment: The systemic nature of lupus makes Lupus Nephritis more complex to treat than isolated kidney conditions. Physicians must manage kidney inflammation and address the broader spectrum of lupus symptoms, including joint pain, skin rashes, cardiovascular complications, and neurological symptoms. Treatment regimens often require a multidisciplinary approach involving rheumatologists, nephrologists, and other specialists.

Organ-Specific and Systemic Symptoms: Patients with Lupus Nephritis may experience renal-specific symptoms, such as proteinuria, hematuria, and edema, alongside systemic lupus symptoms like fatigue, joint inflammation, photosensitivity, and fever.

2. Fluctuating Disease Activity (Flares and Remissions): Another hallmark of Lupus Nephritis is its unpredictable course, characterized by periods of active disease (flares) and relative inactivity (remissions).

Flares: During flares, patients may experience a sudden worsening of kidney function, with increased proteinuria, rising creatinine levels, and symptoms such as swelling, high blood pressure, and changes in urine output. Flares can be triggered by factors such as stress, infections, and changes in medication.

Remissions: Between flares, patients may enter periods of remission, during which their kidney function stabilizes, and the inflammatory activity in the kidneys decreases. The goal of treatment in Lupus Nephritis is often to induce remission and prolong the periods of disease inactivity.

Management Challenges: The fluctuating nature of Lupus Nephritis presents a unique challenge in management. Treatment regimens may need to be adjusted during flares to aggressively control inflammation, while long-term maintenance therapy aims to prevent relapses and maintain remission. Monitoring disease activity through regular blood and urine tests is crucial to detect early signs of flares.

Conclusion

In conclusion, Lupus Nephritis differs from other kidney diseases in several ways, particularly its autoimmune etiology, systemic involvement, and fluctuating disease activity. These features make treating it more complex and require a comprehensive approach that addresses kidney-specific symptoms and lupus's broader manifestations. Understanding these differences is essential for guiding appropriate management and improving outcomes for patients with Lupus Nephritis.

Take Home Points

- Lupus Nephritis affects 40-60% of lupus patients, causing kidney inflammation.
- The disease involves systemic immune dysfunction, impacting multiple organs.
- It follows a course of flares and remissions, making management challenging.
- Early detection and regular monitoring are critical to prevent long-term kidney damage.
- Treatment focuses on controlling the immune response and preserving kidney function.

References

1. Tsokos GC. Systemic lupus erythematosus. N Engl J Med. 2011;365(22):2110-21.
2. D'Cruz DP, Khamashta MA, Hughes GR. Systemic lupus erythematosus. Lancet. 2007;369(9561):587-96.
3. Rahman A, Isenberg DA. Systemic lupus erythematosus. N Engl J Med. 2008;358(9):929-39.

4. Haque S, Bruce IN. Therapy insight: systemic lupus erythematosus as a risk factor for cardiovascular disease. Nat Clin Pract Cardiovasc Med. 2005;2(8):423-30.
5. Willerson JT, Ridker PM. Inflammation as a cardiovascular risk factor. Circulation. 2004;109(21 Suppl 1):II2-10.
6. Zeller CB, Appenzeller S. Cardiovascular disease in systemic lupus erythematosus: the role of traditional and lupus related risk factors. Curr Cardiol Rev. 2008;4(2):116-22.
7. Hannah JR, D'Cruz DP. Pulmonary Complications of Systemic Lupus Erythematosus. Semin Respir Crit Care Med. 2019;40(2): 227-34.
8. Shin JI, Lee KH, Park S, Yang JW, Kim HJ, Song K, et al. Systemic Lupus Erythematosus and Lung Involvement: A Comprehensive Review. J Clin Med. 2022;11(22).
9. Kamen DL, Strange C. Pulmonary manifestations of systemic lupus erythematosus. Clin Chest Med. 2010;31(3):479-88.
10. Amarnani R, Yeoh SA, Denneny EK, Wincup C. Lupus and the Lungs: The Assessment and Management of Pulmonary Manifestations of Systemic Lupus Erythematosus. Front Med (Lausanne). 2020;7:610257.
11. Huong DL, Papo T, Beaufils H, Wechsler B, Bletry O, Baumelou A, et al. Renal involvement in systemic lupus erythematosus. A study of 180 patients from a single center. Medicine (Baltimore). 1999;78(3):148-66.
12. Lichtnekert J, Anders HJ. Lupus nephritis-related chronic kidney disease. Nat Rev Rheumatol. 2024;20(11):699-711.
13. Ota Y, Srinivasan A, Capizzano AA, Bapuraj JR, Kim J, Kurokawa R, et al. Central Nervous System Systemic Lupus Erythematosus: Pathophysiologic, Clinical, and Imaging Features. Radiographics. 2022;42(1):212-32.
14. Sciascia S, Bertolaccini ML, Baldovino S, Roccatello D, Khamashta MA, Sanna G. Central nervous system involvement in systemic lupus erythematosus: Overview on classification criteria. Autoimmun Rev. 2013;12(3):426-9.
15. Font J, Ramos-Casals M, Cervera R, Garcia-Carrasco M, Torras A, Siso A, et al. Cardiovascular risk factors and the long-term outcome of lupus nephritis. QJM. 2001;94(1):19-26.
16. Waldman M, Appel GB. Update on the treatment of lupus nephritis. Kidney Int. 2006;70(8):1403-12.

CHAPTER 3

EARLY SIGNS AND SYMPTOMS

LEARN TO RECOGNIZE THE EARLY CLUES FROM YOUR BODY

Abstract

This chapter explores the early signs and symptoms of lupus nephritis through Leah's personal journey, offering patients an emotional and relatable entry point into understanding this serious condition. It highlights common symptoms such as profound fatigue, swelling, changes in urine, skin rashes, and joint pain. Emphasis is placed on the subtlety and variability of symptoms, the risks of delayed diagnosis, and the importance of early recognition. Practical tables and explanations guide readers in identifying warning signs. By blending personal storytelling with clear medical education, the chapter empowers patients to seek timely intervention and protect their kidney health.

Keywords: Fatigue, Swelling (Edema), Proteinuria, Early Detection, Patient Awareness

Each morning, Leah woke not to the promise of a new day but to a body that felt like it was betraying her from within. Sleep no longer refreshed her; instead, she awoke even more exhausted than when she had collapsed into bed the night before. Her body felt heavy, every muscle aching under an invisible weight. The simple act of sitting up demanded a strength she no longer possessed.

The swelling in her feet became her first adversary of each day. She would sit on the edge of her bed, staring at them, willing the tightness and throbbing to ease. Her once-favorite morning ritual — slipping on her sneakers and taking her dog for a peaceful walk through the neighborhood — now felt like a cruel test. Each step was a battle between her spirit's determination and her body's resistance.

But it wasn't just the physical exhaustion. It was a deep, bone-aching weariness, a relentless fog that dulled her mind and blurred her days. Attending her college classes, once a source of pride and excitement, became an ordeal. Concentrating on lectures or discussions felt like trying to read through a thick mist. Even holding a pen felt taxing. Leah began to dread the simplest tasks — not because they were intellectually challenging, but because her body felt utterly unprepared to meet the world each day.

Her hands, once agile and expressive, betrayed her too. Stiff and swollen each morning, they resisted the commands she gave them. Typing an assignment, holding a coffee cup, even tying her hair into a simple ponytail became small daily battles against an unseen enemy. Each task completed was a small victory overshadowed by the fear that tomorrow might be even harder.

Every morning, the mirror confronted her with new betrayals. The rash across her cheeks and nose, once faint and ignorable, grew darker, angrier. It became impossible to cover with makeup, impossible to explain away. Leah lingered longer at her reflection, seeing a stranger — tired, inflamed, a version of herself slipping further from the girl she used to be.

Weeks passed, and the symptoms only multiplied. What truly terrified her was the change in her urine — dark, frothy, and ominously different. At first, Leah told herself it was nothing, maybe dehydration. But deep inside, a quiet dread grew. She could no longer silence it.

Multiple visits to doctors and emergency rooms followed, each appointment filled with tests, each ending with more questions than answers. Finally, one day, her world shifted.

The doctor sat her down and, with quiet compassion, told her: *"Leah, you have lupus. And it's affecting your kidneys."*

Lupus nephritis. Two words she had never heard before, now carrying the weight of everything she had been feeling. The swelling, the exhaustion, the fog, the rashes, the foamy urine — all interconnected signs of her own immune system waging war against her kidneys.

Leah sat in stunned silence, trying to absorb the news. The fear, the helplessness, the betrayal she felt by her own body — it was overwhelming. She realized that what she had been trying to push through was not something temporary. It was something serious. Something that would require every ounce of courage she had.

Leah's story is not unique.

For many patients with systemic lupus erythematosus, lupus nephritis doesn't arrive loudly. It sneaks in through exhaustion, swelling, and minor signs that are easy to dismiss. And often, by the time the symptoms become undeniable, the kidneys are already under attack.

Fatigue, joint pain, rashes — these early signs are often mistaken for simple stress, allergies, or overwork. However, subtle changes in urine color, persistent swelling, and an escalation of symptoms must never be ignored.

Early recognition is not just important — it is life-saving. Timely intervention can mean the difference between preserving kidney function and facing a lifetime of dialysis or transplant.

In the following sections, we will explore these warning signs in greater detail — not to create fear, but to empower. With knowledge comes hope. And with hope, like Leah, patients can learn to fight back — and reclaim their futures.

Understanding Early Signs of Lupus Nephritis

Early detection of lupus nephritis can be challenging, as the symptoms may be subtle. However, some specific signs and symptoms can suggest the involvement of the kidneys in lupus (1). The symptoms specific to lupus nephritis are given in Table 3.

Table 3: Symptoms of Lupus Nephritis

Symptoms of Lupus Nephritis	Description
Edema/Swelling	Swelling can occur in different body areas, especially in the legs, ankles, and around the eyes, often because of fluid (salt and water) retention.
Changes in Urine Output	Changes in frequency of urination, along with possible variations in the color or smell of the urine.
Proteinuria	Finding excess protein in urine during tests can be a sign of kidney damage. This presents as foamy urine.
Hematuria	The appearance of blood in the urine can lead to a reddish or pinkish hue.
Hypertension	High blood pressure is often seen in lupus nephritis and can lead to further decline in kidney function.

1. Swelling or Edema:

Swelling, particularly in the lower legs, ankles, feet, and around the eyes, indicates fluid retention, suggesting kidney involvement in conditions like lupus. The swelling occurs because the kidneys are not functioning optimally and struggle to balance salt and water. When the kidneys fail to remove excess salt and water from the blood, it accumulates in the tissues, leading to noticeable swelling.

This type of swelling is often more pronounced at the end of the day or after long periods of sitting or standing, primarily due to gravity pulling fluids down in the legs when upright. People might notice that their shoes feel tighter than usual, have to increase the belt size at the waist, or that rings or watches become uncomfortably snug. Swelling around the eyes, often noticed upon waking, can also be a symptom and may be particularly distressing due to its visible impact.

Such fluid retention causes discomfort and can exacerbate other symptoms, such as increased blood pressure and stress on the heart. It's essential for individuals experiencing this type of swelling to seek medical attention, as it can be a sign of worsening kidney function or an indication that their current treatment needs adjustment.

Managing this symptom often involves lifestyle changes such as reducing salt intake, which can help decrease fluid retention. Additionally, doctors may prescribe diuretics called "water pills" that help the kidneys eliminate excess fluid. Elevating the legs when sitting and avoiding standing for prolonged periods can also help reduce swelling. Regular monitoring and treatment adjustments are crucial to manage this condition effectively and prevent further complications associated with fluid overload. However, all these methods are temporary, and it is essential to see a kidney doctor who can diagnose and treat Lupus Nephritis.

2. Changes in Urination:

Observing changes in urine is crucial for detecting underlying kidney issues, and several key characteristics can offer important insights into the health. When the urine becomes frothy, foamy, or bubbly, this is typically a sign of proteinuria, an abnormal amount of protein in the urine. Proteinuria is often a direct indication of kidney damage because healthy kidneys usually prevent large molecules like proteins from passing into the urine. When the kidneys are damaged, this filtering system breaks down, allowing proteins to escape into the urine, creating a frothy appearance due to the protein mixing with air when the urine hits the water in the toilet. This is like the froth seen at the top of the milkshake due to protein in the milk.

Additionally, changes in urine color can significantly indicate health issues. If urine appears darker than usual or has a red tint, this may suggest the presence of blood, a condition known as hematuria. This symptom is particularly concerning because it indicates that there may be bleeding within the urinary tract or kidneys, which could be due to inflammation, infection, or damage to these organs.

Changes in the frequency of urination, whether an increase or decrease, can also signal kidney problems. An increased frequency might suggest the body is attempting to rid itself of excess waste or fluid due to the kidneys' impaired ability to filter blood properly. On the other hand, a decrease in urination might indicate that the kidneys are not producing as much urine as they should, which can be a sign of worsening kidney function or severe dehydration.

It's important for individuals noticing these changes to consult with a healthcare provider. Regular monitoring and proactive management of these symptoms are key to maintaining kidney health and preventing complications in patients with lupus.

3. High Blood Pressure:

Increased blood pressure, often silent in its early stages, is a common complication of impaired kidney function. The kidneys play a pivotal role in regulating blood pressure by controlling fluid balance and releasing hormones that influence blood pressure. When the kidneys are damaged, their ability to manage these functions diminishes, leading to increased blood pressure, known as hypertension. This rise in pressure is particularly insidious because it typically does not cause noticeable symptoms early on, making it easy to overlook without regular monitoring.

Hypertension is a significant concern for individuals with kidney issues because high blood pressure can cause further harm to the kidneys. It can exacerbate the damage to the renal arteries, worsening kidney function in a detrimental cycle where damaged kidneys lead to higher blood pressure, which then causes more kidney damage. This relationship underscores the importance of regular blood pressure monitoring, especially for those known to have or are at risk for kidney disease.

Detection typically occurs during routine health check-ups, where a simple blood pressure test can reveal higher-than-normal readings. If high blood pressure is identified, it is crucial to manage it effectively to prevent additional kidney damage and reduce the risk of other severe complications like heart disease and stroke.

Managing hypertension in the context of kidney impairment usually involves a combination of lifestyle adjustments and medication. Lifestyle changes may include adopting a heart-healthy diet, reducing sodium intake, maintaining a healthy weight, engaging in regular physical activity, limiting alcohol consumption, and avoiding smoking.

Regular follow-up with healthcare providers is essential to monitor the effectiveness of the treatment plan and adjust as needed. This proactive approach helps manage both blood pressure and the overall health of the kidneys, aiming to slow the progression of kidney damage and reduce the risk of cardiovascular disease.

Symptoms of Lupus Nephritis may vary between individuals

The symptoms of lupus nephritis can differ quite a bit from person to person due to the complex nature of systemic lupus erythematosus and its unique impact on each individual. Some may face severe symptoms like noticeable swelling in the legs, ankles, and around the eyes or changes in urination such as blood or foamy urine due to protein leakage. On the other hand, some individuals might only notice mild fatigue or slight swelling, which can make early detection more challenging. These differences can affect how quickly the disease is diagnosed and treated.

Various factors, including the severity of lupus, existing health issues, and even genes, can shape the symptoms of lupus nephritis. For instance, some people might mainly deal with joint pain and skin rashes related to lupus, while kidney issues remain undetected until routine lab tests reveal them. In contrast, others may notice early kidney symptoms like high blood pressure or swelling without the more common signs of lupus, such as the butterfly rash on the face. This variety underscores the importance of personalized monitoring and care for lupus patients, as kidney involvement can progress in many ways.

Additionally, the unpredictable nature of lupus itself adds to the variability of symptoms. Lupus nephritis can flare up, leading to worsened symptoms during active disease, followed by periods of remission where symptoms may lessen or even vanish. This ebb and flow can make it challenging to anticipate the severity and timing of kidney-related symptoms, highlighting the need for regular check-ups and tailored treatment strategies that cater to each patient's unique experience with lupus nephritis (1, 2).

Common misdiagnoses and delays in recognizing Lupus Nephritis

Lupus nephritis is often misdiagnosed or recognized late because its early symptoms can easily be mistaken for less serious conditions. Challenges in early diagnosis and misinterpretations of Lupus Nephritis are given in Table 4.

Table 4: Challenges in Early Diagnosis and Misinterpretations of Lupus Nephritis

Key issues	Explanation	Common Misinterpretations
Early Symptoms Overlap	Symptoms such as fatigue, joint pain, swelling, and changes in urination are often seen in various conditions, which can make it challenging to recognize lupus nephritis in its early stages.	Urinary tract infections, stress-related fatigue, dehydration
Misdiagnosis of Protein in Urine	Proteinuria (the presence of protein in urine) is frequently confused with less serious issues, such as temporary kidney stress or dehydration, mainly when frothy or foamy urine is the sole indicator.	Vigorous exercise, dehydration
Misinterpretation of Swelling	Swelling in the legs or around the eyes might be seen as just a little fluid retention or possibly related to heart concerns.	High salt intake, mild heart issues

Variability in Symptom Presentation	Some patients might experience symptoms of systemic lupus, like rashes and joint pain, even when there aren't clear signs of kidney involvement, which can shift the attention towards the non-renal features of lupus.	Non-kidney-focused lupus treatment
Fluctuating Symptom Patterns	Lupus nephritis can have ups and downs, with symptoms getting worse at times and then improving, which can sometimes create the misunderstanding that everything is fine during the remission period.	The belief that the condition is resolved during symptom-free periods

Common signs such as fatigue, joint pain, swelling, and changes in urination can overlap with many other ailments, including urinary tract infections, stress-related fatigue, or even dehydration. The subtlety and variability of these symptoms make it challenging for patients and healthcare providers to consider lupus nephritis, especially if a person hasn't been previously diagnosed with systemic lupus erythematosus. This delay in identifying lupus nephritis can worsen kidney function before initiating proper treatment.

One of the most frequent misdiagnoses in lupus nephritis cases involves mistaking proteinuria (protein in the urine) for benign conditions, such as transient kidney stress from vigorous exercise or dehydration due to menstrual bleeding or urinary tract infection. Frothy or foamy urine, often a sign of protein leakage should be investigated thoroughly before attributing to these non-serious causes, even if the patient is otherwise asymptomatic. Similarly, swelling in the legs or around the eyes may be dismissed as fluid retention due to high salt intake or mild heart issues. Without a comprehensive assessment, these early signs of kidney involvement are often overlooked, allowing the disease to progress silently.

Another factor contributing to delayed diagnosis is the variability in how lupus nephritis presents itself. Some patients may exhibit more systemic lupus symptoms, such as skin rashes, joint pain, or fatigue, without any noticeable kidney-related symptoms. In such cases, the focus may remain on managing these signs of lupus while kidney damage continues undetected. On the other hand, kidney-specific symptoms like high blood pressure or changes in urination might be mistaken for primary kidney diseases, leading to treatments that do not address the underlying autoimmune cause.

Additionally, lupus nephritis can flare intermittently, with symptoms worsening and then subsiding, creating periods where the disease appears dormant. During these remission phases, symptoms may decrease or disappear, leading patients and healthcare providers to believe the issue has been resolved. This fluctuating nature can further complicate diagnosis, as it is easy to underestimate the seriousness of the condition when symptoms are not constant. Regular monitoring of kidney function in lupus patients, even during remission periods, is critical to catching lupus nephritis early before it leads to irreversible damage.

Overall, the complexity of lupus nephritis, combined with the overlap of symptoms with other common conditions, contributes to frequent misdiagnoses and delays in proper treatment. Raising awareness among healthcare providers and patients about the specific signs of kidney involvement in lupus is essential for ensuring earlier recognition and intervention. Timely diagnosis and treatment can help preserve kidney function, prevent further damage, and improve long-term outcomes for those with lupus nephritis.

Conclusion

Lupus nephritis is more than a complication of lupus—it is a serious condition that can silently damage the kidneys if not recognized and treated early. Unlike other kidney diseases, it arises from the immune system's misdirected attack, leading to unpredictable cycles of flares and remissions. Leah's journey shows how subtle symptoms can quickly escalate, and why early detection, regular monitoring, and timely treatment are essential. With knowledge, proactive care, and support, patients can protect kidney function and continue to live meaningful, fulfilling lives.

Take home points

- Almost half of people with lupus get kidney problems.
- Lupus nephritis is kidney inflammation caused by lupus.

- It comes in flares and remissions, so it can be unpredictable.
- Regular check-ups help catch problems early.
- Treatment aims to protect your kidneys and keep them working.

References

1. Musa R, Brent LH, Qurie A. Lupus Nephritis. StatPearls. Treasure Island (FL) 2024.
2. Crosslin KL, Wiginton KL. The impact of race and ethnicity on disease severity in systemic lupus erythematosus. Ethn Dis. 2009;19(3):301-7.

CHAPTER 4

HOW DOCTORS DETECT LUPUS NEPHRITIS

SEE HOW TESTS AND SCANS GUIDE DIAGNOSIS

Abstract

This chapter explores the critical process of diagnosing lupus nephritis, weaving Leah's emotional journey with a clear explanation of key diagnostic tools. It highlights the importance of early detection through careful history-taking, physical examination, urinalysis, blood tests, complement levels, imaging studies, and kidney biopsy. Each diagnostic step is explained in patient-friendly language, helping readers understand how lupus can silently attack the kidneys and why timely intervention matters. By empowering patients with knowledge about the signs, tests, and interpretations, this chapter lays the foundation for effective treatment planning and offers hope for preserving long-term kidney health.

Keywords: Urinalysis**,** Kidney Biopsy**,** Proteinuria**,** Early Detection**,** Immune Markers

After weeks of struggling with exhaustion, swelling, and unsettling changes in her body, Leah finally sat across from her doctor, searching his face for answers. She listened carefully as he gently explained that her symptoms pointed to something serious — possibly lupus and, more worryingly, lupus nephritis, a condition where lupus causes inflammation and damage to the kidneys. Leah felt her heart pound harder as he spoke, each beat echoing her rising fear. She had always trusted her body to heal itself, but now it seemed her body was waging a secret war she barely understood.

The days that followed became a blur of tests. First came the detailed review of her medical history. Sitting stiffly in the sterile exam room, Leah tried to recall everything — any family history of autoimmune diseases, past infections, medications she had taken, strange symptoms she had brushed off. She remembered that a few family members had autoimmune conditions, but none had faced anything quite like this. As the doctor gently probed deeper — asking about unexplained fevers, weight loss, and high blood pressure — Leah realized just how many quiet warnings she had ignored.

Next came the urinalysis. It seemed so simple — just a small sample in a plastic cup. Yet a few hours later, the results carried a heavy truth: Leah's urine contained high levels of protein, a sign that her kidneys were leaking precious proteins instead of holding them in. The frothiness she had seen swirling in the toilet was no coincidence — it was her body's cry for help. Worse still, small amounts of blood were detected in her urine, a stark signal that inflammation was already damaging her kidneys' delicate filters.

Blood tests followed each vial a window into the turmoil inside her. Her creatinine and blood urea nitrogen (BUN) levels were elevated, showing that her kidneys were struggling to clear waste. Tests for her immune system revealed a storm raging inside her: positive antinuclear antibodies (ANA) and elevated anti-double-stranded DNA (anti-dsDNA) levels, classic hallmarks of lupus attacking her tissues.

Despite all the mounting evidence, her doctor explained they needed one more test — the most definitive—a kidney biopsy. Leah's heart clenched at the thought. The idea of a needle piercing her side to take a piece of her kidney felt overwhelming, almost too much to bear. But the doctor's calm reassurance and her growing determination gave her courage. She wanted answers. She needed to fight.

The next day, Leah found herself lying still in the radiology suite, the cool ultrasound gel pressed against her back. The procedure blurred into a haze of local anesthesia and sedating medications. Though she doesn't remember every detail, she does remember clutching the hand of a kind nurse who whispered encouragement as the needle found its mark.

When the biopsy results arrived, Leah braced herself. Sitting once again in the doctor's office, she listened as he explained she had Class IV lupus nephritis—a severe form involving widespread inflammation and damage across many parts of her kidneys. The words felt heavy, landing on her chest like stones. Tears welled in her eyes, not from weakness but from the weight of knowing that life as she knew it had changed.

But even amid the fear, the doctor's words carried hope. There were treatments. Powerful ones. With aggressive therapy, they could quiet the storm in her kidneys, prevent further destruction, and preserve the life she still had ahead of her. She was not powerless. She was not alone,

In the upcoming sections, this chapter will examine the diagnostic tests used to identify lupus nephritis. Grasping these diagnostics is essential to the patient's journey with lupus nephritis.

Importance of Early Diagnosis

Lupus nephritis happens when systemic lupus erythematosus affects the kidneys, leading to inflammation that hampers their vital role in filtering waste and extra fluids from the blood. In this condition, the immune system, which typically defends the body against infections, mistakenly targets healthy kidney tissues, particularly the fragile glomeruli, the filtering unit of the kidney. This inflammation can interfere with the kidneys' ability to filter properly, resulting in proteins and blood cells leaking into the urine, often one of the initial signs of lupus nephritis.

It's crucial to catch lupus nephritis early because, if it's not addressed, the inflammation can cause lasting damage to the kidneys, affecting their function over time. If left untreated, lupus nephritis may advance to more serious kidney issues, such as chronic kidney disease or kidney failure, which could necessitate dialysis or a transplant. Regular tests like urinalysis and blood work are needed for timely diagnosis of lupus nephritis. This allows your doctor to start treatment for Lupus Nephritis in a timely to reduce inflammation, slow the disease's progression, and protect kidney function. Early intervention, including immunosuppressive medications, which can dampen the overactive immune system, can prevent irreversible damage and improve long-term outcomes for lupus nephritis patients.

Initial Evaluation

The diagnostic process for lupus nephritis is critical in ensuring appropriate management and treatment. It usually starts with a comprehensive evaluation of the patient's medical history and a thorough physical examination. During this initial phase, healthcare providers focus on identifying any clinical manifestations that might suggest lupus, including but not limited to systemic symptoms such as joint pain, skin rashes, and general fatigue, which are common in lupus patients.

A. Detailed Patient History

The first step in diagnosing lupus nephritis is a thorough and detailed review of the patient's medical history, which is a foundation for understanding the broader context of their symptoms. This process involves gathering information about past medical issues, chronic conditions, and the onset and duration of new or ongoing symptoms. Patients are asked about their family medical history, particularly any relatives with autoimmune diseases, as this can increase their risk of conditions like systemic lupus erythematosus or lupus nephritis. Additionally, healthcare providers inquire about current and past treatments or medications, as certain drugs or therapies can influence symptoms or mask signs of underlying disease or trigger symptoms of lupus. Understanding the patient's overall health and medical background allows doctors to identify patterns pointing toward lupus nephritis. It helps differentiate it from other potential causes of kidney dysfunction or systemic symptoms.

During the medical history review, doctors specifically focus on symptoms commonly associated with lupus, as these can serve as key indicators. Joint pain is a frequent symptom, often presenting as stiffness or swelling, particularly in the morning, which may indicate lupus-related inflammation. Your doctor will also ask about any new skin rash, with particular attention to the butterfly-shaped rash that appears across the cheeks and nose and any rash that worsens with sun exposure. Fatigue is another common symptom that doesn't improve with rest and can be an early sign of both systemic lupus and lupus nephritis. While common in lupus, these symptoms can be subtle or develop gradually, so a detailed and careful medical history is essential. By gathering this information, your doctors can better assess the likelihood of lupus nephritis and determine the need for further diagnostic testing, such as urine and blood tests, to confirm the diagnosis and evaluate the extent of kidney involvement (1, 2).

B. Family and Personal Medical History:

Alongside assessing the patient's current symptoms, your doctor will ask for a thorough family medical history. Autoimmune diseases like lupus and lupus nephritis can have a genetic link, which means that those with a family member with a diagnosis of systemic lupus erythematosus, rheumatoid arthritis, or other autoimmune disorders are more likely to develop lupus or lupus nephritis themselves. Almost 10% of individuals with lupus have a family member diagnosed with the condition, and first-degree relatives face a greater risk of developing autoimmune diseases compared to the general population (3, 4). Medical providers can evaluate the patient's genetic risk by asking about lupus, kidney disease, or similar autoimmune issues in close family members. This information is essential for understanding the overall context of the patient's health and the possibility that their symptoms might point to lupus nephritis or another autoimmune condition. Even if lupus hasn't been officially diagnosed in the family, a history of autoimmune symptoms—like unexplained joint pain, ongoing fatigue, or skin problems—can offer valuable insights into potential genetic risk factors (5).

The family medical history not only aids in identifying potential genetic risks but also helps guide further diagnostic investigations. For instance, if a close relative has been diagnosed with lupus or kidney disease, the healthcare provider may prioritize specific tests, such as urinalysis or kidney function tests, to rule out or confirm lupus nephritis. Additionally, understanding the family history can help doctors recognize patterns of disease presentation that might not be immediately apparent through symptoms alone. For example, a patient with a family history of lupus might exhibit early, subtle signs of kidney involvement that could be overlooked. This more profound understanding of the patient's familial health background enables more proactive and targeted diagnostic strategies, helping to detect lupus nephritis at an earlier stage when treatment interventions can most effectively prevent long-term kidney damage.

C. Physical Examination

During the physical examination, healthcare providers will carefully assess the patient for any physical signs that could indicate lupus or lupus nephritis. One important sign of lupus is the malar rash, often called the butterfly-shaped rash, which appears across the nose and extends to both cheeks. This rash can vary in intensity and may become more pronounced with sun exposure, a common condition known as photosensitivity in lupus patients. Besides the malar rash, the medical providers will also check for other skin conditions, such as discoid rashes—round, red, scaly patches that can leave scars and are frequently seen in those with lupus. These rashes typically appear on areas of the skin that are exposed to sunlight, like the face, neck, and arms, making a thorough skin examination crucial for diagnosing lupus (6-9).

In addition to looking at skin symptoms, healthcare providers will also take a close look at the joints for any signs of swelling, tenderness, or stiffness, which are common in lupus and may suggest inflammation in the joints, known as inflammatory arthritis. This joint pain can often be more intense in the morning and might affect several joints, restricting movement. The medical providers will gently examine the joints to check for warmth or fluid buildup, indicating inflammation (10, 11). Your doctor will look in your mouth for any sores in the mouth, which can be a sign of lupus, they will look for any lumps in the neck armpits to look for swollen lymph nodes, a marker of active inflammation in the body.

While lupus nephritis might not always present clear external signs, swelling in the lower legs, particularly around the ankles, feet, or eyes, or in the belly could signal fluid retention related to kidney problems. The physical exam will also involve checking blood pressure, as high blood pressure is a frequent complication of lupus nephritis when the kidneys are impacted. Your doctor will listen to your lungs via stethoscope to see if there is any fluid accumulation in the lungs. By carefully assessing the skin, joints, and other physical indicators, the doctors collect valuable information to help determine or exclude lupus nephritis, guiding the next steps in the diagnostic process (11-13).

D. Urine Changes:

Changes in urine can often be one of the early signs of lupus affecting the kidneys. If the patient notices frothy or foamy urine, it might be a sign of proteinuria, which happens when proteins that usually remain in the blood leak into the urine due to damage in the kidneys' filtering units called glomeruli. Excess protein in the urine is a significant indicator of kidney issues, suggesting that the kidneys aren't effectively filtering waste or wasting essential proteins in the urine. Additionally, if the patients find blood in their urine, known as hematuria, it could indicate inflammation or damage to the kidneys' filtering structures, allowing red blood cells to enter the urine. Both proteinuria and hematuria can occur without any noticeable symptoms, making them crucial markers for spotting lupus nephritis. Changes in urine color, like a darker or reddish hue, can also signify kidney involvement due to bleeding or significant inflammation (11, 14, 15).

In addition to changes in urine composition, variations in urination frequency and volume are important signs of kidney involvement in lupus nephritis. The patient might notice that they need to urinate more frequently, especially at night, or that their urine output is unusually large or small. A decrease in urine output, known as oliguria, can signal serious kidney dysfunction, suggesting that the kidneys are struggling to maintain a normal balance of fluids and waste.

These urinary changes may start subtle but can become more pronounced as the disease progresses, emphasizing the need for early detection. If the patient observes these changes, medical providers typically recommend further diagnostic tests like urinalysis to check for proteins, blood, or other irregularities in the urine.

E. Review of Symptoms

This initial consultation might also involve a detailed discussion of any recent symptoms that could suggest an exacerbation or advancement of lupus nephritis, such as increased leg swelling, high blood pressure, or a recent increase in fatigue. This comprehensive approach helps doctors determine whether lupus nephritis could be present and what further tests are needed to confirm the diagnosis.

By methodically gathering this information, healthcare providers can assess the likelihood of lupus nephritis and decide on the appropriate next steps in the diagnostic process, such as lab tests and potentially a kidney biopsy, to confirm the presence and extent of kidney involvement. This careful and detailed evaluation is essential for creating an effective and tailored treatment plan for patients suspected of having lupus nephritis.

Laboratory Tests

 # Urine Tests:

A routine urine test, known as a urinalysis, is typically one of the first diagnostic steps taken when lupus nephritis is suspected. This simple yet crucial test provides valuable information about the health of the kidneys by detecting abnormalities in the urine that may indicate kidney damage.

What Urinalysis Checks For:

1. Protein in urine (Proteinuria): Healthy kidneys usually filter waste from the blood while retaining essential components like proteins. When the kidneys are damaged, however, they may fail to keep these proteins in the blood, allowing them to leak into the urine. The presence of protein in the urine, a condition known as proteinuria, is a significant indicator of kidney impairment. High protein levels in the urine can suggest that the kidney's filtering units, glomeruli, are damaged.

2. Blood in urine (Hematuria): Under normal circumstances, urine shouldn't have any blood in it because healthy kidneys filter out waste while keeping blood cells in the bloodstream. When blood is present in the urine, a condition called hematuria occurs, pointing to potential issues in the urinary tract, including kidney problems. In cases of lupus nephritis, hematuria might suggest inflammation or damage to the kidney's filtering units. These glomeruli can become more permeable, allowing red blood cells to leak into the urine. Often, this blood isn't visible to the naked eye and can only be seen under a microscope, known as microhematuria. Although subtle, microhematuria is an important sign of kidney involvement, often indicating early inflammation or damage before more serious symptoms arise. Detecting this early through routine urinalysis is essential, as it enables prompt action to reduce inflammation and protect the kidneys from further harm.

How Urinalysis Is Conducted

The urine test, or urinalysis, is easy and non-invasive to gain important information about kidney health and overall bodily function. It starts with providing a small urine sample in a sterile container and then sent to a lab for thorough analysis. In the lab, the sample will be examined through various tests to identify abnormalities that might suggest health concerns, such as kidney disease, infections, or systemic conditions like lupus nephritis (16).

1. Physical appearance: The first step is to look at the urine's physical appearance, which can provide quick insights into possible issues. The color and clarity are especially important. For instance, very pale or clear urine might mean the person is drinking too much water. On the other hand, dark urine could indicate dehydration or the presence of blood or other unusual substances. If the urine is cloudy, it might suggest an infection or extra proteins. Additionally, urine with a reddish or brownish hue could point to hematuria or blood in the urine, which might signal kidney involvement.

2. Chemical examination: Next, a chemical examination using dipstick strips that have been specially treated is performed. These strips are briefly dipped into the urine sample and change color when they come in contact with specific substances in the urine. This allows the lab to quickly spot the presence of proteins, glucose, ketones, blood, and other compounds. Detecting protein in the urine, known as proteinuria, is especially significant in conditions like lupus nephritis, as it indicates that the kidneys may not be functioning properly. The dipstick test also helps identify other issues, such as elevated sugar (glucose) levels, which could suggest diabetes or ketones produced when fat is metabolized and may indicate uncontrolled diabetes or malnutrition.

3. Microscopic examination: A microscopic examination is performed by placing a small urine sample under a microscope to check for specific cells in the urine. When the kidney functions normally, nothing is present in the urine, and the laboratory technician will not see anything under the microscope. However, sometimes red blood cells can be seen, which suggests hematuria or white blood cells, often indicative of an infection or inflammation. The microscope may also reveal casts—tiny tube-shaped structures made from proteins in the kidney's tubules. The type of casts can provide hints about kidney damage or inflammation. Additionally, the presence of crystals could signal the development of kidney stones. Altogether, these microscopic observations give us valuable insights into the patient's kidneys and urinary system, aiding in diagnosing conditions like lupus nephritis and informing further treatment options.

Why It's Important

Conducting a urinalysis is a fast and affordable way to check for kidney diseases, making it a vital tool for the early detection of lupus nephritis. Spotting abnormalities early on can significantly enhance how medical providers manage the condition, potentially slowing its progression and leading to better patient outcomes. If any irregularities are found in the initial urinalysis, additional tests, such as more comprehensive blood tests and possibly a kidney biopsy, might be suggested to confirm the diagnosis and evaluate the level of kidney damage.

 # Blood Tests:

Blood tests are a critical component in diagnosing and managing lupus nephritis. These tests provide essential information about kidney function and the immune system's activity, helping physicians determine the extent of the disease and monitor its progression.

1. Assessing Kidney Function:

Creatinine: This byproduct from muscle metabolism is usually filtered from the blood by the kidneys. A blood test that measures creatinine levels is a common way to evaluate kidney function. If creatinine levels in the blood are higher than normal, it may suggest that the kidneys aren't filtering blood as well as they should, which can be a sign of kidney disease.

Blood Urea Nitrogen (BUN): Urea nitrogen is another waste product formed from the breakdown of proteins, which healthy kidneys filter out of the blood. Like creatinine, high levels of BUN can suggest reduced kidney function. However, BUN levels can also be influenced by dehydration or a high-protein diet, so it is usually measured in conjunction with creatinine.

2. Identifying Autoimmune Activity:

Lupus nephritis is an autoimmune condition where the body's immune system attacks the kidneys. Specific blood tests help diagnoses lupus and identify markers of autoimmune activity:

A. Antinuclear Antibodies (ANA): A. One of the most frequently used tests is the Antinuclear Antibodies (ANA) test. This test identifies antinuclear antibodies, immune proteins that mistakenly target the nuclei of the body's cells. Finding ANA in the blood is a key indicator of lupus, as most individuals will test positive for it. However, a positive ANA test isn't exclusive to lupus or lupus nephritis and can also appear in other autoimmune disorders. While a positive ANA result strongly suggests the possibility of an autoimmune condition, it typically isn't sufficient on its own to confirm a lupus nephritis diagnosis. Instead, it acts as a starting point for further exploration. Doctors often use the ANA result as a cue to perform additional, more specific tests that can help confirm lupus nephritis, especially when kidney involvement is suspected. After identifying a positive ANA, further tests to detect more specific antibodies can assist in tailoring treatment strategies based on the severity and nature of the immune response (17-19).

B. Anti-double-stranded DNA (anti-dsDNA) Antibodies: Another important test is the Anti-double-stranded DNA (anti-dsDNA) antibodies test, which detects antibodies that target double-stranded DNA within cells. Unlike ANA, which can be found in various autoimmune conditions, anti-dsDNA antibodies are much more closely linked to lupus and are strongly associated with lupus nephritis. Patients with kidney involvement often have high levels of anti-dsDNA antibodies, making their presence a key indicator of disease activity. The higher the levels of these antibodies in the blood, the more likely it is that lupus is affecting the kidneys and causing inflammation. Keeping track of anti-dsDNA antibody levels over time can also provide valuable insights into disease progression or treatment response. Rising levels may signal an impending flare while decreasing levels suggest that treatment effectively manages the immune response. Thus, the anti-dsDNA test plays a crucial role in diagnosing lupus nephritis, guiding treatment choices, and monitoring the success of interventions to reduce kidney inflammation (20, 21).

Why These Tests Matter

Together, these blood tests offer a thorough insight into kidney health and the immune system's status for patients with lupus. When creatinine and BUN levels are elevated, it indicates potential kidney function issues, which may lead to further evaluations and possibly more proactive management strategies to avert additional harm. Additionally, identifying autoimmune markers such as ANA and anti-dsDNA is essential for confirming a lupus diagnosis, evaluating its severity, and informing treatment choices.

Regularly monitoring these blood tests is vital for individuals with lupus nephritis. It allows for adjustments in treatments aimed at reducing immune system activity, preventing kidney damage, and effectively managing symptoms. This proactive strategy can greatly enhance outcomes and improve the quality of life for those facing this challenging condition.

 # Complement Levels:

Complement proteins play a vital role in our immune system as part of a protective network that safeguards the body from infections and helps remove damaged cells. These proteins work alongside immune cells to detect and eliminate harmful invaders like bacteria and viruses while also clearing away unnecessary cells. Additionally, complement proteins initiate inflammation, the body’s natural response to injury or infection, facilitating tissue repair and healing. However, in autoimmune diseases like lupus, the immune system can mistakenly target healthy tissues, leading to inappropriate activation of complement proteins. Instead of defending against infections, they can attack the body's cells, including the kidneys, resulting in excessive consumption of these proteins. There are multiple complement proteins in our blood. However, there are two complement proteins that are commonly tested, known as C3 and C4 complement proteins.

In the case of lupus nephritis, where lupus directly impacts the kidneys, complement proteins C3 and C4 are depleted rapidly in the blood due to ongoing inflammation and kidney damage. The kidneys, which filter waste and excess fluid from the blood, are particularly susceptible to this immune attack; the more active the lupus, the more complement proteins are consumed. Thus, medical providers monitor these complement levels through blood tests. Usually, low C3 and C4 levels indicate heightened lupus activity. When C3 and C4 levels drop, it suggests that the immune system is active and mistakenly targeting the kidneys, causing inflammation and potentially leading to kidney damage. This decrease in complement levels offers important insights into the severity of inflammation and the risk of further kidney harm.

A reduction in complement levels often signals a lupus flare, indicating increased disease activity. In lupus nephritis, this flare can result in kidney inflammation, making it crucial to monitor complement levels closely. Regularly testing these proteins allows doctors to assess disease activity and determine if the current treatment is working effectively to decrease the inflammation. If complement levels continue to decline, it may indicate active disease and the need for change in treatment plan to prevent kidney damage. Conversely, if complement levels start to normalize, it suggests that the treatment is successfully decreasing immune activity and aiding kidney recovery. Healthcare providers can proactively address potential flare-ups and safeguard kidney function by tracking these changes.

In summary, keeping a close eye on complement levels through regular testing provides crucial insights into lupus activity and aids in guiding treatment decisions. By diligently monitoring these proteins, healthcare providers can help stabilize lupus, prevent flares, and protect the kidneys from further harm, ultimately improving long-term outcomes for individuals with lupus nephritis. This proactive approach is essential for maintaining kidney function and overall health in lupus patients (22-26).

 # Imaging Tests:

Imaging tests are an important support tool in diagnosing and managing lupus nephritis, even though they aren't the main method for diagnosis. These tests are especially helpful in examining the condition of the kidneys, allowing medical providers to identify any structural issues that may be causing the symptoms and ruling out other possible reasons for kidney problems.

Role of Imaging Tests in Lupus Nephritis

1. Assessment of Kidney Size and Structure: Imaging tests can offer valuable insights into the size of the kidneys, which is crucial since notably smaller kidneys might indicate chronic, irreversible damage. Additionally, any changes in the kidney's structure, like thickening or thinning of the tissues, can be detected and tracked over time.

2. Ruling Out Other Conditions: Besides checking for signs of lupus nephritis, imaging tests can help identify other kidney issues that may resemble or complicate lupus nephritis, like blockages, tumors, or stones. Addressing these conditions might involve different management approaches or treatments.

Common Imaging Tests Used

1. Ultrasound: This is the most frequently used imaging test in the context of lupus nephritis for several reasons:

Non-invasive and Safe: Ultrasound uses sound waves to create images of the kidneys. It does not involve radiation, making it safe for repeated use, which is particularly important for monitoring chronic conditions like lupus nephritis.

Cost-Effective and Widely Available: It is relatively inexpensive compared to other imaging modalities and is available in most hospital settings.

Diagnostic Insights: Ultrasound can show abnormalities in the shape and size of the kidneys and can detect other kidney problems that might coexist with lupus nephritis, such as hydronephrosis (kidney swelling due to a build-up of urine).

2. CT scan (Computed Tomography): Provides a clearer picture and can be helpful when ultrasound results are unclear or when a more detailed view of the anatomy is needed for diagnosis or treatment planning. However, CT scans involve radiation exposure and can be quite costly.

3. MRI (Magnetic Resonance Imaging): Offers detailed, high-resolution images of the kidneys and nearby tissues without radiation, making it particularly helpful in complex cases requiring a closer look at tissue integrity. However, MRI can be costly, and not all hospitals can perform these scans.

Kidney Biopsy:

A kidney biopsy is regarded as the gold standard for diagnosing lupus nephritis. All patients who are suspected to have lupus nephritis from history, physical exam, urine, and blood tests need a kidney biopsy to make the diagnosis of lupus nephritis. This procedure involves the extraction of a small piece of kidney tissue for detailed examination, providing invaluable insights into the cause, extent, and nature of the damage caused by the disease.

The Process of Kidney Biopsy

A kidney biopsy is usually done with local anesthesia, allowing patients to remain awake while the area around their kidneys is numbed, which helps keep discomfort to a minimum. This method is less invasive than surgeries requiring general anesthesia, leading to quicker recovery times and a reduced risk of complications.

Before the procedure, the patient is comfortably positioned on their stomach or side, giving the doctor easy access to the kidneys, which are located in the lower back. The doctors use imaging techniques like ultrasound or CT scans to guide the biopsy needle accurately toward the kidney. These tools provide real-time visuals of the kidney, ensuring precise needle placement while minimizing the risk of damage to nearby organs and tissues. Once the kidney is located, a specialized biopsy needle is gently inserted through the skin to collect a small core of kidney tissue. Imaging guidance is crucial for the procedure's success, helping to target the correct area of the kidney while avoiding important structures like blood vessels. By carefully following this method, healthcare providers can safely obtain the necessary tissue sample for diagnosis while keeping the risk of complications, such as bleeding, to a minimum. The kidney biopsy is done in only one kidney usually determined by the doctor doing the procedure depending on the images of the kidneys. The disease due to lupus nephritis affects both kidneys equally, so it does not matter which kidney is biopsied. The whole process of kidney biopsy typically takes 15-20 minutes. Your doctor will closely observe your blood pressure and heart rate 2-4 hours after the procedure.

Examination and Analysis

After a kidney tissue sample is taken during a biopsy, it’s sent to a histopathology lab for analysis. A specialist called a pathologist, trained to identify diseases by examining tissues and cells, examines the sample under a microscope. This detailed inspection is key to understanding the kidney changes linked to lupus nephritis. The pathologist looks for specific signs of damage caused by the immune system mistakenly attacking the kidneys. This thorough examination provides insights that blood tests or imaging alone can’t offer, helping to confirm the diagnosis and assess the severity of the disease.

In lupus nephritis, the immune system's attack on the kidneys results in swelling and damage in the kidney's filtering units, known as glomeruli. The presence of inflammation indicates that the immune system is actively harming the kidneys, disrupting their ability to filter waste from the blood. The pathologist evaluates the presence of inflammation in the kidney. They also examine the severity of the inflammation. This guides kidney doctors and rheumatologists in determining the treatment plan for Lupus Nephritis. Severe inflammation suggests an aggressive disease that requires prompt attention to prevent further kidney damage.

The pathologist looks for scarring, or fibrosis, in the kidney tissue. Scarring occurs when inflammation causes lasting damage, replacing healthy kidney tissue with scar tissue that can't perform the kidneys' normal functions. The amount of scarring helps doctors gauge how much permanent damage has been done and whether the disease has progressed to a more serious stage, like chronic kidney disease.

The pathologist also searches for immune complexes, clusters of antibodies, and antigens. These immune complexes are a hallmark of lupus nephritis and form when the immune system mistakenly attacks the body's tissues. In lupus, these complexes can become trapped in the kidney's filtering units, leading to further inflammation and damage. Identifying these immune complexes under the microscope confirms that the kidney damage is due to lupus. The pathologist also notes how much of the tissue is affected by these immune complexes, helping doctors understand the activity of the disease and guiding treatment decisions.

In summary, examining the kidney tissue provides essential insights into inflammation, scarring, and immune complexes, which assist doctors in evaluating the severity of lupus nephritis and determining the appropriate treatment. This comprehensive analysis is vital for accurate diagnosis and effective disease management.

How to interpret the Kidney Biopsy and Importance of Biopsy Findings

The kidney biopsy confirms the presence of lupus nephritis and helps classify it into different categories, each with its severity level. These categories, or classes, range from mild to severe forms of lupus nephritis, and the findings in each class guide medical providers in choosing the best treatment approach and understanding the likely outcomes or prognosis for the patient (Table 1).

Table 1: Classes of Lupus Nephritis

Classes of Lupus Nephritis	Description	Symptoms	Treatment Approach
Class I: Minimal Mesangial Lupus Nephritis	Mildest form; kidneys function normally; only minor microscopic changes.	Typically, none may be detected through biopsy.	Less aggressive due to normal kidney function. Needs treatment to prevent severe flare of Lupus Nephritis
Class II: Mesangial Proliferative Lupus Nephritis	Slight increase in cells in the mesangial area; mild disease; often no noticeable symptoms.	Usually none; may require monitoring for inflammation.	Careful monitoring requires treatment to prevent progression and prevent severe flares of Lupus Nephritis.
Class III: Focal Proliferative Lupus Nephritis	Significant inflammation and damage to some glomeruli	Blood or protein in urine, swelling, high blood pressure.	Aggressive immunosuppressive treatment to decrease inflammation and preserve kidney function
Class IV: Diffuse Proliferative Lupus Nephritis	Significant inflammation in many glomeruli, impairing kidney filtration; serious symptoms.	Blood or protein in urine, swelling, high blood pressure, impairment of kidney function	Aggressive immunosuppressive treatment to decrease inflammation and preserve kidney function
Class V: Membranous Lupus Nephritis	Thickening and holes in the walls of glomeruli leading to large amounts of proteinuria and	Swelling, protein leakage, and potential worsening of kidney function.	Immunosuppressive treatment to decrease the deposits and holes in the glomeruli walls, manage proteinuria, and prevent kidney damage

Class VI: Advanced Sclerosis Lupus Nephritis	Worst form of Lupus Nephritis as this signifies scarring in the kidney and no active inflammation in the kidney	Swelling, protein in urine, abnormal kidney function	No need for immunosuppressive treatment; treatment to slow down the progression of scarring in the kidneys

Class I: Minimal Mesangial Lupus Nephritis is the mildest form of lupus nephritis. The kidneys function normally in this class; only minor changes can be seen under a microscope. Most people with this form may not experience noticeable symptoms related to their kidney health, and the disease is often only detected through a biopsy. Because kidney function remains normal, treatment is less aggressive than in more severe forms of lupus nephritis and focused on preventing severe flares of lupus nephritis.

Class II: Mesangial Proliferative Lupus Nephritis shows an increase in the number of inflammatory cells in a part of the kidney/glomeruli called the mesangial area, which filters blood and removes waste. This mild disease may not lead to noticeable symptoms, and kidney function often remains normal. However, the increase in cells is a sign of inflammation, which may require careful monitoring and treatment to decrease scarring in the kidney and prevent severe flares.

Class III: Focal Proliferative Lupus Nephritis and **Class IV: Diffuse Proliferative Lupus Nephritis** represent the most severe forms of the disease. In these classes, there is significant inflammation and damage to the glomeruli, the tiny filters in the kidneys responsible for cleaning the blood. Class III affects parts of glomeruli, **while Class IV** involves damage to the whole glomeruli. This damage can impair the kidneys' ability to filter waste effectively, leading to more noticeable symptoms, such as high serum creatinine, blood or protein in the urine, swelling, and high blood pressure. Class III and IV lupus nephritis require aggressive immunosuppressive treatment to decrease the inflammation in the kidney and prevent further damage and loss of kidney function.

Class V: Membranous Lupus Nephritis is characterized by a thickening of the walls and the development of tiny holes in the walls of the glomeruli, the filtering units of the kidneys. The thickening of the glomeruli walls is due to the deposition of antigen-antibody complexes, which then cause damage to the cells, causing tiny holes. This thickening and development of tiny holes leads to a leakage of protein into the urine, a condition called proteinuria. When large amounts of protein are lost through the urine, it can cause other health problems, such as low protein levels in the blood, high cholesterol levels in the blood, and swelling in the legs and feet, and if left untreated, will lead to worsening kidney function. Class V lupus nephritis requires immunosuppressive treatment to decrease the deposition of antigen-antibody complexes in the glomeruli, leading to decreased protein in urine and reducing the risk of long-term kidney damage.

Class VI: Advanced Sclerosis Lupus Nephritis is characterized by scarring in the kidney tissue and no active inflammation in the kidney. This is usually seen as a sequel to previous flares of lupus nephritis, either untreated or not adequately treated. Once there is advanced scarring in the kidney, usually immunosuppressive medications are not needed as there is no active inflammation. The goal of treatment is geared towards slowing the scarring and progression of chronic kidney disease.

Each class of lupus nephritis has different levels of severity and implications for treatment. The biopsy findings help guide doctors in determining the appropriate therapies to control the inflammation and protect kidney function while providing insight into the long-term prognosis (11, 27-30).

Guiding Treatment Decisions

The detailed information from a kidney biopsy helps doctors tailor treatment strategies more effectively. For example, patients with class III, IV, and V of lupus nephritis often require aggressive treatment to decrease inflammation, prevent irreversible kidney damage, and preserve kidney function. Treatment may include immunosuppressive drugs to reduce the immune system's activity and prevent further damage to kidney tissues (31).

Conclusion

Diagnosing lupus nephritis can feel overwhelming, but each test plays an important role in uncovering how lupus affects the kidneys. From simple urine and blood tests to the more detailed kidney biopsy, these steps provide doctors with the information needed to choose the best treatment plan. Early detection is key — the sooner lupus nephritis is identified, the greater the chance of protecting kidney function and preventing long-term damage.

Take home points

- Early diagnosis helps protect your kidneys.
- A detailed history and exam give doctors important clues.
- Urine and blood tests show early signs of kidney damage.
- Low complement levels signal active lupus nephritis.
- A kidney biopsy confirms the diagnosis and guides treatment.

References

1. Emorinken A, Dic-Ijiewere MO, Erameh CO, Ugheoke AJ, Agbadaola OR, Agbebaku FO. Clinical and laboratory profile of systemic lupus erythematosus patients at a rural tertiary centre in South-South Nigeria: experience from a new rheumatology clinic. Reumatologia. 2021;59(6):402-10.
2. Justiz Vaillant AA, Goyal A, Varacallo M. Systemic Lupus Erythematosus. StatPearls. Treasure Island (FL)2024.
3. Wong M, Tsao BP. Current topics in human SLE genetics. Springer Semin Immunopathol. 2006;28(2):97-107.
4. Walters HM, Pan N, Moorthy LN, Ward MJ, Peterson MG, Lehman TJ. Patterns and influence of familial autoimmunity in pediatric systemic lupus erythematosus. Pediatr Rheumatol Online J. 2012;10(1):22.
5. Ashournia P, Sadeghi P, Rezaei N, Moradinejad MH, Ziaee V. Prevalence of Family History of Autoimmune Disorders in Juvenile Systemic Lupus Erythematosus. Maedica (Bucur). 2018;13(1):21-4.
6. Fijalkowska A, Kadziela M, Zebrowska A. The Spectrum of Cutaneous Manifestations in Lupus Erythematosus: A Comprehensive Review. J Clin Med. 2024;13(8).
7. Patel P, Werth V. Cutaneous lupus erythematosus: a review. Dermatol Clin. 2002;20(3):373-85, v.
8. Stull C, Sprow G, Werth VP. Cutaneous Involvement in Systemic Lupus Erythematosus: A Review for the Rheumatologist. J Rheumatol. 2023;50(1):27-35.
9. Werth VP. Clinical manifestations of cutaneous lupus erythematosus. Autoimmun Rev. 2005;4(5):296-302.
10. Santacruz JC, Mantilla MJ, Pulido S, Isaza JR, Tuta E, Agudelo CA, et al. A Practical Overview of the Articular Manifestations of Systemic Lupus Erythematosus. Cureus. 2023;15(9):e44964.
11. Musa R, Brent LH, Qurie A. Lupus Nephritis. StatPearls. Treasure Island (FL)2024.

12. Taylor EB, Ryan MJ. Understanding mechanisms of hypertension in systemic lupus erythematosus. Ther Adv Cardiovasc Dis. 2016; 11(1):20-32.
13. Choe JY, Park SH, Kim JY, Jung HY, Kim SK. A case of systemic lupus erythematosus presenting as malignant hypertension with hypertensive retinopathy. Korean J Intern Med. 2010;25(3):341-4.
14. Saxena R, Mahajan T, Mohan C. Lupus nephritis: current update. Arthritis Res Ther. 2011;13(5):240.
15. Chedid A, Rossi GM, Peyronel F, Menez S, Atta MG, Bagnasco SM, et al. Low-Level Proteinuria in Systemic Lupus Erythematosus. Kidney Int Rep. 2020;5(12):2333-40.
16. Queremel Milani DA, Jialal I. Urinalysis. StatPearls. Treasure Island (FL)2024.
17. Pisetsky DS, Lipsky PE. New insights into the role of antinuclear antibodies in systemic lupus erythematosus. Nat Rev Rheumatol. 2020;16(10):565-79.
18. Pisetsky DS. Evolving story of autoantibodies in systemic lupus erythematosus. J Autoimmun. 2020;110:102356.
19. Nashi RA, Shmerling RH. Antinuclear Antibody Testing for the Diagnosis of Systemic Lupus Erythematosus. Med Clin North Am. 2021;105(2):387-96.
20. Rojo R, Calvo Alen J, Prada A, Valor S, Roy G, Lopez-Hoyos M, et al. Recommendations for the use of anti-dsDNA autoantibodies in the diagnosis and follow-up of systemic lupus erythematosus - A proposal from an expert panel. Autoimmun Rev. 2023;22(12): 103479.
21. Infantino M, Nagy E, Bizzaro N, Fischer K, Bossuyt X, Damoiseaux J. Anti-dsDNA antibodies in the classification criteria of systemic lupus erythematosus. J Transl Autoimmun. 2022;5:100139.
22. Walport MJ. Complement and systemic lupus erythematosus. Arthritis Res. 2002;4 Suppl 3(Suppl 3):S279-93.
23. Bao L, Cunningham PN, Quigg RJ. Complement in Lupus Nephritis: New Perspectives. Kidney Dis (Basel). 2015;1(2):91-9.
24. Birmingham DJ, Hebert LA. The Complement System in Lupus Nephritis. Semin Nephrol. 2015;35(5):444-54.
25. Bao L, Quigg RJ. Complement in lupus nephritis: the good, the bad, and the unknown. Semin Nephrol. 2007;27(1):69-80.
26. Weinstein A, Alexander RV, Zack DJ. A Review of Complement Activation in SLE. Curr Rheumatol Rep. 2021;23(3):16.
27. Markowitz GS, D'Agati VD. Classification of lupus nephritis. Curr Opin Nephrol Hypertens. 2009;18(3):220-5.

28. Parikh SV, Almaani S, Brodsky S, Rovin BH. Update on Lupus Nephritis: Core Curriculum 2020. Am J Kidney Dis. 2020;76(2): 265-81.
29. Stokes MB, D'Agati VD. Classification of Lupus Nephritis; Time for a Change? Adv Chronic Kidney Dis. 2019;26(5):323-9.
30. Weening JJ, D'Agati VD, Schwartz MM, Seshan SV, Alpers CE, Appel GB, et al. The classification of glomerulonephritis in systemic lupus erythematosus revisited. Kidney Int. 2004;65(2):521-30.
31. Kuhn A, Bonsmann G, Anders HJ, Herzer P, Tenbrock K, Schneider M. The Diagnosis and Treatment of Systemic Lupus Erythematosus. Dtsch Arztebl Int. 2015;112(25):423-32.

CHAPTER 5

TREATMENTS THAT HELP

EXPLORE OPTIONS THAT PROTECT AND HEAL YOUR KIDNEYS

Abstract

This chapter offers a friendly and detailed look at treating lupus nephritis, focusing on a well-organized two-phase strategy: induction and maintenance. In the induction phase, the goal is to quickly reduce kidney inflammation with high-dose corticosteroids and immunosuppressants like mycophenolate mofetil cyclophosphamide, along with newer options such as voclosporin and belimumab. After achieving remission, the maintenance phase involves using lower doses of therapies to prevent relapse while reducing long-term side effects. Additionally, the chapter highlights non-immunosuppressive treatments like hydroxychloroquine, ACE inhibitors/ARBs, and diuretics, emphasizing their importance in protecting the kidneys. It also showcases patient-centered approaches and personalized treatment plans, reflecting the ongoing evolution of care for lupus nephritis.

Keywords: Lupus Nephritis, Immunosuppressants, Induction Therapy, Maintenance Phase

After being diagnosed with lupus nephritis, Leah met with the nephrologist, a doctor who specializes in kidney diseases—sitting in the hospital bed, her mind swirling with uncertainty. She feels overwhelmed, not having heard of lupus nephritis before, and her thoughts race with questions about what this diagnosis means for her future. When she finally meets the nephrologist, her anxiety deepens, but she hopes for answers.

The nephrologist explains that while lupus nephritis is a serious condition, well-established treatment options can help manage the disease and protect her kidneys from further damage. Leah listens carefully, trying to process the information, as the doctor describes a two-phase approach to treatment.

The first phase, the induction phase, is designed to aggressively suppress the inflammation causing her kidneys to malfunction. It's explained to her as an urgent, critical step—like putting out a fire. Strong medications such as high-dose corticosteroids and immunosuppressants, which suppress the immune system, are needed to bring the disease under control quickly. Leah hears the words "strong medications," and her concern grows. The nephrologist acknowledges this and cautions her that while these medications are powerful and necessary, they also carry potential side effects that need careful management and monitoring.

Leah nods as the doctor describes the second phase, the maintenance phase. Once the lupus nephritis is under control, she will enter this phase. The goal here is to keep the disease in control, i.e., remission, to prevent it from flaring up again, and to use lower doses of medications. The nephrologist reassures her that this phase is less intense, allowing for a better balance between managing side effects and protecting her kidneys. Lily feels slightly relieved, knowing this phase will be more manageable in the long-term.

Over the next few months, Leah embarks on her journey through the induction phase. Her healthcare team closely monitors her progress, adjusting her medications and keeping an eye on the side effects. The high-dose corticosteroids begin to take their toll, causing weight gain and mood swings. Leah struggles with these changes but knows her symptoms are slowly improving. She understands that this aggressive approach is only temporary and that her long-term health is the priority.

As Leah begins to see the improvement in her condition, she takes comfort in the care she receives, knowing that her journey through lupus nephritis is guided by a well-structured plan to protect her kidneys and overall well-being.

Managing lupus nephritis focuses on controlling the underlying lupus activity and safeguarding the kidneys from additional harm. This chapter delves into the different treatment options available for lupus nephritis, such as immunosuppressants, non-immunosuppressive therapies, and new and emerging treatments.

Treatment of Lupus Nephritis

The treatment of Lupus Nephritis is based on the findings on the kidney biopsy and class of Lupus Nephritis found on the kidney biopsy. The details of the class of kidney biopsy are discussed in the previous chapter, "Diagnosis of Lupus Nephritis."

Treatment of Class I, II, and VI lupus nephritis is primarily based on slowing down scarring in the kidney and preventing flares of Lupus Nephritis. Class I, II, and VI lupus nephritis do not have significant inflammation in the kidney and, hence, do not need immunosuppressive medications. However, all patients with class I, II, and VI Lupus Nephritis should be on hydroxychloroquine. Hydroxychloroquine has been shown to prevent further flare of lupus nephritis. These patients should also be on medications called angiotensin convertase inhibitors or angiotensin receptor blockers (ACE-i/ARB) to decrease the protein in the urine and slow down the scarring in the kidney.

The treatment for class III, IV, and V lupus nephritis should include immunosuppressants to decrease the inflammation in the kidney, along with hydroxychloroquine and angiotensin convertase inhibitors/angiotensin receptor blockers. The treatment is usually divided into two phases for class III, IV, and V lupus nephritis: the induction and maintenance phases (1) (Figure 1). Understanding these phases can help to see how treatment for lupus nephritis is carefully planned to manage the disease effectively over time.

Induction Phase (6-12 months) **(Glucocorticoids + immunosuppressants + Hydroxychloroquine + ACE-i/ARB) to treat LN and decreases the inflammation in the kidney**	***Maintenance Phase (36 months)*** **(Lower dose of immunosuppressants + hydroxychloroquine + ACE-i/ARB) to prevent subsequent flare of LN**

Figure 1: Two-phase approach in treating Lupus Nephritis

A. Induction Phase:

The induction phase is the first step in treatment. The goal of the induction phase is to treat the disease. This aggressive phase aims to quickly control the active inflammation in the kidneys and the body. It's like putting out a fire; the goal is to rapidly calm the immune system to stop it from attacking the kidneys. The medications used during this phase are stronger and work quickly. This phase typically lasts about 6- 12 months, depending on the severity of the symptoms and severity of the disease. At the end of the induction phase, the Lupus Nephritis should be in remission, which means that the inflammation in the kidney should be reduced to minimal or none.

Medications Used in Induction:

1. High-dose corticosteroids (like prednisone) quickly reduce inflammation.
2. Cyclophosphamide
3. Mycophenolate mofetil (MMF)
4. Voclosporin
5. Belimumab
6. Obinutuzumab
7. Combination of the above medications

These are all powerful immunosuppressant drugs that help suppress the immune system and prevent it from causing damage to the kidneys.

All Lupus Nephritis patients should always be on hydroxychloroquine and ACE-i/ARB during the induction phase.

B. Maintenance Phase:

After the induction phase, when lupus nephritis is in remission, i.e., the inflammation in the kidney is reduced to minimal or none, then the maintenance phase begins. This phase focuses on preventing the flare of lupus nephritis and keeping the disease in remission. Since the goal is primarily to prevent further flares, the dose of immunosuppressants is much lower than in the induction phase. This phase should last at least 3 years.

Medications Used in Maintenance:

1. Mycophenolate mofetil (MMF) (lower dose than induction phase)
2. Azathioprine

All Lupus Nephritis patients should always be on hydroxychloroquine and ACE-i/ARB during the induction phase.

Why Both Phases Are Important:

1. Induction phase: Stopping Immediate Damage The induction phase quickly controls the disease, preventing it from causing immediate and severe kidney damage.

2. Maintenance Phase Long-term Control: The maintenance phase helps keep the disease under control over the long term, preventing it from flaring up again and causing more damage to the kidneys

Balancing Treatment and Side Effects: Starting with more potent treatments helps quickly get symptoms under control while switching to less intense treatments helps minimize side effects over the long term.

Understanding these phases helps the patients to see why different medications are used at various times to treat lupus nephritis. It's all about finding the right balance between controlling the disease and managing side effects to maintain good health and quality of life.

 # Immunosuppressants:

Immunosuppressants are the cornerstone of therapy for lupus nephritis because they help reduce the activity of the immune system, thereby preventing it from attacking the kidneys.

A. Corticosteroids:

Prednisone and similar corticosteroids are commonly used as initial treatments for conditions like lupus nephritis due to their potent anti-inflammatory effects and ability to suppress the immune system rapidly. These medications mimic the effects of natural hormones produced by the adrenal glands, which reduce inflammation and modulate the immune response. This makes them very effective in controlling symptoms of lupus nephritis, such as swelling and pain, and preventing the immune system from causing further kidney damage (2-4).

Benefits of Corticosteroids:

1. Rapid Relief: Corticosteroids can quickly decrease inflammation in the kidneys and other organs like skin and joints, significantly relieving rash, joint pain, and swelling.

2. Immunosuppression: Steroids help suppress the immune system by decreasing the function of immune cells in the body, which is crucial in treating autoimmune conditions lke lupus, where the body's immune system attacks its tissues.

Side Effects of Long-Term Use:

While corticosteroids are highly effective in managing inflammation and controlling autoimmune activity in lupus nephritis, long-term use can lead to several side effects. These effects underscore the importance of careful management, close monitoring, and using the lowest effective dose for the shortest possible duration (5-8). Below are some of the key side effects associated with prolonged corticosteroid therapy (Table 1):

Table 1: Side effects of corticosteroids and management of those side effects

Side Effect	Details	Management
Weight Gain and Metabolic Changes	• Increased appetite • Altered fat, protein, and carbohydrate processing • Insulin resistance and diabetes.	• Dietary counseling is needed to manage weight and metabolic issues. • Regular monitoring for steroid-induced diabetes.
Increased Risk of Infections	• Bacterial, viral, and fungal infections • Opportunistic infections like pneumonia and Pneumocystis jirovecii pneumonia (PJP)	• Regular monitoring • Vaccination • Prophylactic treatments
Bone Density Loss (Osteoporosis)	• Decreases calcium/phosphate absorption • Increases bone resorption • Leading to brittle bones • Increased fracture risk.	• Calcium and vitamin D supplements • Medications like bisphosphonates • Regular bone density scans (DEXA) for early detection.

Side Effect	Details	Management
Mood and Psychological Effects	• Mood swings • Anxiety • Irritability • Depression • Steroid-induced psychosis	• Close monitoring of mental health • Psychological support • Medications for mood stabilization.
High Blood Pressure (Hypertension)	• Sodium and water retention • Elevating blood pressure • Increasing cardiovascular risk.	• Blood pressure monitoring • Low-sodium diet • Antihypertensive medications.
Diabetes and Glucose Intolerance	• Insulin resistance • Worsening of pre-existing diabetes.	• Regular blood sugar monitoring • Adjustments to diabetes management plans.
Ulcers in stomach	• Irritation of the lining of the stomach and duodenum	• Medications to decrease acid production in the stomach, like proton pump inhibitors (pantoprazole) or histamine -2 blockers (famotidine)
Skin Changes	• Thinning skin • Increased bruising • Slower wound healing • Stretch marks • Increased facial hair growth (hirsutism)	• Skincare • Regular monitoring for skin-related complications
Eye problems	• Cataracts • Glaucoma	• Regular eye exams

1. Weight Gain and Metabolic Changes: Corticosteroids often increase appetite and alter how the body processes fats, proteins, and carbohydrates, frequently leading to weight gain. This is not just a result of increased caloric intake but also changes in the body's fat distribution. Patients may notice fat accumulating around the abdomen, face (sometimes called "moon face"), and upper back ("buffalo hump"). These changes can be distressing, impacting self-esteem and overall well-being, especially for long-term users.

Metabolic Impact: Corticosteroids can cause insulin resistance, which may lead to steroid-induced diabetes. This is particularly concerning for patients with lupus nephritis because diabetes can further affect kidney function.

Increased Appetite: Managing diet while on corticosteroids can be challenging due to a significantly increased appetite. Medical providers often recommend dietary counseling to help mitigate weight gain and metabolic complications.

2. Increased Risk of Infections: Corticosteroids suppress the immune system, which, while beneficial in controlling autoimmune diseases, also makes the body more vulnerable to infections. Patients on long-term corticosteroid therapy have a higher risk of bacterial, viral, and fungal infections, some of which can become severe or life-threatening.

Opportunistic Infections: Long-term use can make patients susceptible to infections like pneumonia, urinary tract infections, and rare, opportunistic infections such as Pneumocystis jirovecii pneumonia (PJP), which can be severe.

Monitoring: Due to the increased infection risk, regular monitoring, vaccination (where appropriate), and early detection of symptoms are crucial. Patients may also need prophylactic antibiotics, as well as antiviral or antifungal medications, depending on their risk level.

3. Bone Density Loss (Osteoporosis): One of the most concerning long-term side effects of corticosteroids is osteoporosis, a condition where bones become weak and brittle. Corticosteroids interfere with the bone-rebuilding process by decreasing the absorption of calcium and phosphate and increasing bone resorption, leading to a net loss of calcium from the bones and a decrease in bone density.

Increased Risk of Fractures: Prolonged corticosteroid use leads to weak bones and is associated with a higher risk of fractures, particularly in the spine and hips, even from minimal trauma.

Prevention and Management: Your doctor will recommend calcium and vitamin D supplements to prevent calcium loss from the bones. In some cases, medications like bisphosphonates may be prescribed to help strengthen bones. Regular bone density scans (DEXA scans) are essential for early detection and management of osteoporosis in long-term corticosteroid users.

4. Additional Side Effects: Beyond the more visible and severe complications, corticosteroids can cause a wide range of additional side effects that affect various aspects of physical and mental health:

Mood and Psychological Effects: Long-term corticosteroid use is known to cause mood swings, anxiety, irritability, and even depression. In some cases, patients may experience more severe psychiatric symptoms, such as steroid-induced psychosis, characterized by confusion, hallucinations, or delusions. Managing these mental health effects is often as important as managing the physical side effects.

High Blood Pressure (Hypertension): Corticosteroids can cause the body to retain sodium and water, leading to elevated blood pressure. This can increase the risk of cardiovascular complications, including heart disease and stroke, particularly in patients with lupus nephritis, who may already be at an elevated cardiovascular risk.

Diabetes and Glucose Intolerance: Corticosteroids can impair insulin function and lead to increased blood sugar levels, sometimes resulting in steroid-induced diabetes. Patients with pre-existing diabetes may find their condition worsens while on corticosteroids, requiring adjustments in their diabetes management plan.

Stomach Ulcers: Corticosteroids cause irritation in the lining of the stomach causing ulcers in the stomach manifesting as pain burning in the chest and upper abdomen area. It can also lead to indigestion, nausea, and vomiting. Your doctor will usually give you medications like proton pump inhibitors (pantoprazole) or H2 blockers (famotidine) to decrease the acid in the stomach and prevent ulcers in the stomach.

Skin Changes: Prolonged corticosteroid use can lead to skin thinning, making it more susceptible to bruising, tears, and slower wound healing. Patients may also notice stretch marks (striae) and increased facial hair growth (hirsutism).

Cataracts and Glaucoma: Long-term corticosteroid use is associated with the development of cataracts (clouding of the lens in the eye) and glaucoma (increased pressure in the eye), which can lead to vision impairment. Regular eye exams are crucial for early detection and treatment.

Managing Side Effects:

Because of the potential side effects associated with long-term corticosteroid use, close medical supervision is essential for anyone on these medications. The following strategies are commonly used to help manage and reduce the impact of these side effects:

1. Regular Monitoring and Dose Adjustments: Frequent follow-up appointments allow medical providers to track developing side effects. By regularly monitoring health indicators, such as bone density or blood pressure, they can adjust corticosteroid dosages to minimize complications while controlling the disease.

2. Supplemental Treatments: Medical providers often recommend additional treatments to counteract specific side effects. For example, calcium and vitamin D supplements are commonly prescribed to help reduce the risk of osteoporosis and support bone health. In some cases, medications may be prescribed to protect against gastric ulcers, a possible consequence of long-term steroid use.

3. Lifestyle Changes: A balanced diet and regular exercise are essential for managing weight gain, maintaining muscle mass, and strengthening bones. Patients may be referred to nutritionists or physical therapists to create individualized plans that support their overall health while minimizing steroid-related side effects. For example, weight-bearing exercises can improve bone density, and a low-sodium diet can help manage blood pressure.

Corticosteroids remain a fundamental part of treating lupus nephritis due to their effectiveness. Despite all the side effects listed above, corticosteroids work well to treat the inflammation in the kidneys and other organs in the body due to lupus. Typically, if you or your loved one has lupus, you already know the benefits of corticosteroids, especially for symptoms of rash, joint pain, and fatigue. However, the goal is to use the lowest dose for the shortest time that controls the disease to minimize potential side effects. The goal is to taper off the corticosteroids as other immunosuppressants can suppress the immune system and have their full impact on the disease. These other immunosuppressants are discussed below.

B. Cyclophosphamide:

Cyclophosphamide is a potent immunosuppressant drug that plays a crucial role in treating severe cases of lupus nephritis, mainly when there is a significant risk of progressing to kidney failure. This medication works by suppressing the immune system to a substantial degree, reducing its ability to attack the body's tissues, including the kidneys. It is one of the strongest immunosuppressants used to treat Lupus Nephritis. It is also one of the oldest and the second medications studied to treat lupus nephritis after corticosteroids. It effectively manages all forms of lupus nephritis, especially the most aggressive type, where other medications may not have been sufficient.

How Cyclophosphamide Works:

Cyclophosphamide belongs to a class of drugs known as alkylating agents, typically used in chemotherapy to treat cancer. It works by interfering with the multiplication of cells, including those of the immune system. By inhibiting the proliferation of these cells, cyclophosphamide reduces the number of immune cells in our body. It decreases the immune response and inflammation in the kidney, helping to prevent further damage to kidney tissues in lupus nephritis (9). The dose of cyclophosphamide used to treat lupus nephritis is lower than the dose typically used to treat cancer.

Use in Lupus Nephritis:

Given its effectiveness, cyclophosphamide is often employed when lupus nephritis is particularly aggressive or rapidly progressing. The goal is to quickly bring the disease under control and prevent the kidneys from failing—a critical situation that would require dialysis or kidney transplantation (10, 11). Cyclophosphamide can be given as oral pills to be taken daily or intravenous infusion every 2-4 weeks. Typically, intravenous infusion uses a total less medication dose and thus is associated with fewer side effects. It is, however, a bit expensive because of the cost of the infusion of the medication in an infusion center.

Potential Side Effects:

Although cyclophosphamide is highly effective in controlling severe lupus nephritis, its potent effects come with the risk of significant side effects. It is crucial for patients undergoing treatment with cyclophosphamide to be closely monitored to manage these risks. Below are some of the most common and serious side effects associated with its use (12-15) (Table 2):

Table 2: Side effects of cyclophosphamide and management of the side effects

Side Effect	Details	Management
Gastrointestinal Effects	• Nausea, vomiting • Loss of appetite	• Anti-nausea medications • Dietary adjustments
Increased Risk of Infections	• Bacterial, viral, and fungal infections • Severe infections like pneumonia, urinary tract infections • Sepsis	• Prophylactic antibiotics, antivirals, or antifungals • Regular monitoring for early infection
Bone Marrow Suppression	• Bone marrow suppression • Anemia • Low white blood cells • Low platelets	• Regular blood tests usually every 2 weeks to monitor white blood cell counts and hemoglobin and platelet count • Medications like filgrastim to stimulate white blood cell production if needed.
Bladder Toxicity	• hemorrhagic cystitis • blood in the urine due to irritation of the lining of the urinary bladder	• Increased oral fluid intake • Intravenous fluid • Mesna (to protect the bladder lining) • Monitoring for early signs of bladder irritation.
Hair Loss (Alopecia)	• Thinning or complete hair loss	• Emotional support • Hair returns once the treatment is completed and lupus nephritis is in remission. Information for patients to manage visible side effects

Side Effect	Details	Management
Increased Risk of Cancer	• Long-term use increases the risk of certain cancers, including bladder cancer and leukemia	• Limit cyclophosphamide use duration • Regular cancer screenings • Plenty of water intake to flush the bladder.
Infertility	• Cyclophosphamide causes damage to dividing cells in the body- and can cause damage to oocytes in females and sperm development in males	• Females: medications like gonadotropin-releasing hormone (GnRH) antagonists induce temporary menopause to protect eggs in ovaries Males: sperm count returns to normal a few months after completion of treatment • Recommend discussion with your kidney doctor about fertility preservation prior to starting cyclophosphamide

1. Increased Risk of Infections: Cyclophosphamide works by suppressing the immune system, which is necessary to prevent it from attacking the kidneys. However, this immune suppression makes the body more vulnerable to infections. Patients on cyclophosphamide may experience severe bacterial, viral, or fungal infections that can sometimes be life-threatening.

Opportunistic Infections: These infections occur more frequently in people with weakened immune systems. Common examples include pneumonia, urinary tract infections, and skin infections. In more severe cases, patients might develop sepsis, a life-threatening condition where the body's response to infection causes widespread inflammation.

Management: Preventive measures often include administering prophylactic antibiotics, antivirals, or antifungal medications. Regular blood tests and monitoring for early signs of infection are also essential.

2. Increased Risk of Cancer: One of the more serious long-term risks of cyclophosphamide use is an increased likelihood of developing certain types of cancer. The drug can damage DNA in rapidly dividing immune and healthy cells.

Bladder Cancer: The risk of bladder cancer is notably higher in patients who receive cyclophosphamide multiple times and for a prolonged duration. The risk of bladder cancer significantly increases in people who smoke cigarettes. So, it is recommended to stop smoking if you smoke if you are or previously received cyclophosphamide.

Leukemia: Some patients may be at risk for secondary leukemia, a form of cancer that arises because of chemotherapy-induced damage to bone marrow cells. However, this risk is low to minimal with the smaller dose of cyclophosphamide used to treat lupus nephritis compared to doses used to treat cancer.

Management: Physicians typically limit the duration of cyclophosphamide use to minimize this risk and may recommend increased cancer screenings, such as regular urine tests to check for blood, which could be an early sign of bladder cancer. Patients may also be advised to drink plenty of water to flush the bladder and reduce irritation.

3. Other Side Effects: In addition to infections and cancer risks, cyclophosphamide is associated with a variety of different side effects, some of which can significantly impact a patient's quality of life:

Hair Loss (Alopecia): One of the more visible and distressing side effects is hair loss. Cyclophosphamide can cause thinning or complete hair loss, often temporary, and hair generally regrows after treatment ends.

Gastrointestinal Effects: Patients may experience nausea, vomiting, or loss of appetite while undergoing treatment with cyclophosphamide. These side effects can usually be managed with anti-nausea medications and dietary adjustments.

Bladder Toxicity: Cyclophosphamide can cause hemorrhagic cystitis, a condition where the lining of the bladder becomes irritated, resulting in blood in the urine (hematuria) and painful urination. This is a direct effect of the drug's metabolites passing through the bladder.

Decreased fertility: Cyclophosphamide interferes with the multiplication of cells; hence, it can cause damage to oocytes (eggs) in ovaries and sperm in men. This is due to the direct effects of cyclophosphamide on the oocytes and sperm. Damage to oocytes can be prevented by causing temporary menopause in females. This temporary menopause causes eggs to go into hibernation and become less prone to damage by cyclophosphamide. The sperm counts usually in men return to pre-treatment level a few weeks to months after completion of treatment with cyclophosphamide.

Managing and Monitoring:

Due to the potentially severe side effects of cyclophosphamide, its use is generally limited to short-term courses. The goal is to minimize harmful effects while achieving control over lupus nephritis. Close monitoring and adjustments are crucial to safely managing this powerful medication. Treatment protocols often include the following strategies:

1. Regular Blood Tests: Frequent blood tests are essential to treatment while on cyclophosphamide. These tests monitor the body's response to the drug and detect any early signs of complications.

White Blood Cell Count: Cyclophosphamide can reduce the production of white blood cells, increasing the risk of infection. Regular blood tests allow medical providers to track white blood cell levels and adjust the dosage if necessary to avoid excessive immune suppression.

Kidney and Liver Function Tests: Since cyclophosphamide can affect the function of vital organs, routine blood tests assess kidney and liver health to ensure the treatment is not damaging these organs.

Monitoring Bone Marrow Function: Blood tests also track the bone marrow's ability to produce blood cells, which cyclophosphamide can affect. Early detection of abnormalities allows for adjustments in treatment before more serious complications arise.

1. Supportive Medications: To help mitigate some of the side effects of cyclophosphamide, medical providers often prescribe additional medications that target specific risks associated with the drug.

Bladder Protection (Mesna): One of the significant concerns with cyclophosphamide is hemorrhagic cystitis, where the bladder lining is irritated, leading to blood in the urine. To prevent this, medical providers may prescribe Mesna, a medication that binds to the toxic byproducts of cyclophosphamide in the bladder, reducing the risk of bladder irritation and bleeding.

Anti-nausea Medications: Cyclophosphamide can cause significant gastrointestinal side effects, including nausea and vomiting. Anti-nausea medications like ondansetron or metoclopramide may be prescribed to help manage these symptoms and improve the patient's quality of life during treatment.

Prophylactic Antibiotics or Antivirals: Due to the increased risk of infections, some patients are prescribed preventive antibiotics or antiviral medications to reduce the likelihood of developing infections such as pneumonia or herpes zoster (shingles).

Gonadotropin-releasing hormone antagonists: To induce temporary menopause in women. This helps prevent the damage to eggs in the ovaries and preserves fertility.

Bone Marrow-Stimulating Agents: In cases where white blood cell counts become critically low, medications such as filgrastim may stimulate the bone marrow to produce more white blood cells, reducing the risk of infection.

2. Follow-Up Care: Close and continuous follow-up care is critical throughout treatment with cyclophosphamide. Regular check-ins with healthcare providers allow for careful adjustments and transitions as the patient progresses through different phases of treatment.

Adjustment of Dosages: As patients respond to treatment, dosages of cyclophosphamide may be adjusted to achieve the best balance between controlling the disease and minimizing side effects. The goal is always to use the lowest effective dose for the shortest duration possible to limit the risks associated with long-term use.

Transition to Maintenance Therapy: Once lupus nephritis is remission, patients are usually transitioned to maintenance therapy for long-term management. This maintenance phase typically involves drugs like mycophenolate mofetil (MMF) or azathioprine, which are effective in maintaining remission.

Monitoring for Long-Term Effects: Long-term monitoring is necessary even after cyclophosphamide treatment ends. The increased risks of cancer, especially bladder cancer, and other side effects may persist, and regular follow-up appointments are essential to detect any complications early.

In summary, cyclophosphamide is an effective treatment option for severe lupus nephritis; its use requires careful consideration of the benefits against the risks and close monitoring for side effects. Its role is often pivotal in cases where rapid control of the disease can prevent irreversible kidney damage and maintain overall kidney function.

C. Mycophenolate Mofetil (MMF):

Mycophenolate Mofetil (MMF) is an essential medication for managing lupus nephritis, particularly for long-term treatment. It is an immunosuppressant that suppresses the immune system and prevents it from attacking the body's tissues, such as the kidneys, in lupus nephritis. MMF is the preferred option for patients with lupus nephritis due to its effectiveness in lupus nephritis, and it is well tolerated with less side effects (16-20). MMF is available as oral pills and used as a twice-a-day medication to be taken 12 hours apart.

How MMF Works:

MMF decreases the proliferation of lymphocytes, a type of white blood cell involved in the immune system. By reducing the number of lymphocytes, MMF lowers the immune system's ability to cause inflammation and damage to the kidneys in patients with lupus nephritis.

Effectiveness and Usage:

MMF is considered as effective as cyclophosphamide in many cases of lupus nephritis, particularly in managing the symptoms and progression of the disease. Due to its efficacy and safety profile, MMF is commonly used as a first-line treatment for lupus nephritis. It also works very well in maintaining disease control over long periods, reducing the frequency and severity of flares (21).

Side Effect Profile:

Mycophenolate Mofetil (MMF) is often favored over cyclophosphamide for long-term management of lupus nephritis due to its relatively milder side effect profile. While MMF is still a potent immunosuppressant and can cause significant side effects, they are generally less severe and more manageable than those associated with cyclophosphamide. Below are some of the most common side effects of MMF and how they can be managed (22-26) (Table 3):

Table 3: Side effects of Mycophenolate and the management

Side Effect	Description	Management
Gastrointestinal Issues	• Diarrhea • Nausea • Vomiting • Abdominal discomfort	• Diarrhea: Adjust the MMF dosage or take it with food. Use anti-diarrheal medications like loperamide if approved. • Nausea/Vomiting: Take smaller doses, use anti-nausea meds like ondansetron, and avoid large meals before MMF
Increased Risk of Infection	• Increase the risk of infections, including upper respiratory, urinary tract, and fungal infections	• Vaccination (e.g., pneumococcal, flu shots), • Prophylactic antibiotics or antivirals
Bone Marrow Suppression	• Anemia • Leukopenia (low white blood cell count) • Thrombocytopenia (low platelet count)	• Regular blood test monitoring • Dose adjustment

1. Gastrointestinal Issues: One of the most frequently reported side effects of MMF involves the gastrointestinal (GI) system, including symptoms like diarrhea, nausea, vomiting, and abdominal discomfort. These symptoms can vary in intensity, but in many cases, they can be managed through dosage adjustments, taking medication with food, or splitting the dose into smaller doses over the day.

Diarrhea: This is a common complaint, but it can often be controlled by adjusting the dosage of MMF or taking the medication with food. Your doctor can check MMF levels in your blood and ensure the levels are not very high. If your doctor approves, some patients can benefit from over-the-counter anti-diarrheal medications like loperamide.

Nausea and Vomiting: These side effects can be mitigated by taking the medication at smaller doses more frequently throughout the day or using anti-nausea medications such as ondansetron. Patients are also advised to avoid eating large meals before taking MMF, which can help ease nausea.

Management and Monitoring: Persistent GI symptoms that don't respond to these strategies may require a more comprehensive assessment, and healthcare providers may adjust the dose or switch to a different formulation of MMF (such as the delayed-release form) to minimize these issues.

2. Increased Risk of Infection: Like other immunosuppressants, MMF suppresses the immune system, reducing the body's ability to fight infections. While the risk of infections is somewhat lower compared to more potent immunosuppressants like cyclophosphamide, it is still a concern, and patients should be closely monitored.

Opportunistic Infections: Patients on MMF may experience upper respiratory infection, urinary tract infection, or fungal infection. More serious infections such as cytomegalovirus (CMV) or pneumocystis pneumonia (PCP), although less common, can occur in severely immunosuppressed patients.

Preventive Measures: Healthcare providers often recommend certain vaccinations before starting MMF, such as the pneumococcal vaccine and flu shot, to reduce infection risk. Sometimes, patients at high risk of infection may be prescribed prophylactic antibiotics or antivirals.

Management: Early recognition of infection symptoms is crucial. Patients are encouraged to seek prompt medical attention if they develop fever, chills, cough, or other signs of infection. Regular blood tests and clinical assessments help to identify infections early, allowing for timely treatment.

3. Potential for Bone Marrow Suppression: MMF can suppress the bone marrow's ability to produce blood cells, leading to anemia, leukopenia (low white blood cell count), or thrombocytopenia (low platelet count). This effect on the bone marrow is one of the reasons patients on MMF require close monitoring through regular blood tests.

Leukopenia: Leukopenia means low white blood cell count. This can increase the risk of infections, making regular monitoring critical. If leukopenia occurs, the dosage of MMF may be adjusted.

Anemia: Anemia means low red blood count. Low red blood cell counts can lead to fatigue, weakness, and other symptoms associated with anemia. Physicians may recommend iron supplements or blood transfusions in more severe cases if the anemia is significant.

Thrombocytopenia: Thrombocytopenia means low platelet cell count in the blood. A reduction in platelets can increase the risk of bleeding and bruising. Patients with thrombocytopenia may need dose adjustments or may require medications that help stimulate platelet production.

Management: Regular complete blood counts (CBC) are essential for early detection of bone marrow suppression. If abnormalities are detected, healthcare providers may lower the MMF dose, temporarily stop the medication, or switch to an alternative therapy to allow the bone marrow to recover.

Long-term Management:

Given its effectiveness and manageable side effects, MMF is an excellent choice for long-term treatment for lupus nephritis. It's essential to regularly monitor the disease activity to adjust dosages as needed and address any potential side effects. This approach helps balance controlling autoimmune activity and minimizing adverse effects, leading to better managing lupus nephritis.

In summary, MMF provides a dependable and relatively safe option for patients with lupus nephritis, effectively managing this complex condition over the long term while controlling side effects.

D. Calcineurin Inhibitors: Tacrolimus and Voclosporin:

Calcineurin Inhibitors are a class of immunosuppressants that are effective in lupus nephritis. This class of medications prevents the white blood cells, especially the lymphocytes, from becoming active, decreasing their function. This class of medicines has four drugs but two of them have been studied in lupus nephritis. These two include Tacrolimus and Voclosporin. Volcosporin is one of the newest medications for the treatment of lupus nephritis and is FDA-approved to treat lupus nephritis. The most important thing to know about this class of medications is that these medications are added to MMF and not used alone. When Voclosporin is added along with MMF to the treatment regimen, there is a greater likelihood to achieve remission and to decrease the dose of corticosteroids much quicker. This strategy helps control lupus nephritis effectively, along with decreasing the side effects of corticosteroids, a major advancement in the field of lupus nephritis in the past 10 years. Both tacrolimus and Voclosporin are available as oral pills to be taken 12 hours apart, once in the morning and once in the evening.

How calcineurin inhibitors work:

Calcineurin inhibitors are immunosuppressants that work by inhibiting calcineurin, an enzyme that activates T-cells (lymphocytes) in the body. This class of medications is very specific in their mechanism of action by inhibiting primarily T- cells. However, in lupus and lupus nephritis, T cells are activated, but there are other immune cells that are activated. Hence, it is mostly used in conjunction with MMF rather than alone.

Advantages of Calcineurin Inhibitors:

The advantage of calcineurin inhibitors is that when used in conjunction with MMF, there is a greater likelihood of achieving remission of lupus nephritis, even with a much lower dose of corticosteroids. Longer use of corticosteroids is associated with higher side effects of infections, diabetes, bone disease, and weight gain. Since Voclosporin is a newer drug, it is one of the few medications which is FDA-approved for the treatment of lupus nephritis. The other difference between tacrolimus and Voclosporin is that tacrolimus levels are usually monitored by your doctor, and the dose is adjusted according to blood levels, but Voclosporin levels do not need to be tested, and a similar dose can be used for everyone without adjusting according to levels.

This class of medications is very effective in decreasing protein in urine and especially effective in patients with Class V lupus nephritis, who present with large amounts of protein in urine.

This new strategy of combination therapy for the treatment of lupus nephritis enables the personalization of a treatment plan for patients with lupus nephritis depending on their clinical presentation, disease activity and kidney biopsy features, rather than giving one immunosuppressant to everyone with lupus nephritis.

Side effects of calcineurin inhibitors:

Calcineurin inhibitors are good medications to control lupus nephritis and decrease inflammation in the kidney due to lupus, but they can increase blood pressure in some people. Close monitoring of blood pressure is needed in patients with calcineurin inhibitors. This class of medications is also associated with a slightly higher risk of diabetes and hyperlipidemia. This risk is lower with the newer medication Voclosporin when compared to tacrolimus. If this group of medications is used for a prolonged time (over 5-10 years), these medications can cause some scarring in the kidney.

Voclosporin is a new medication and, hence, significantly expensive compared to other medications used to treat lupus nephritis. Since it is a new medication, it is not available in all the pharmacies across the country but is only available in specialty pharmacy.

E. Belimumab:

Biologics represent a newer class of treatments in the management of lupus nephritis, with belimumab being one of the prominent examples. These medications work by targeting specific components of the immune system involved in lupus. Belimumab is FDA-approved for treating lupus and lupus nephritis. As with Voclosporin, Belimumab should always be used with MMF to treat lupus nephritis (27-29). Belimumab is given either as an intravenous infusion or subcutaneous self-injections at home.

How Belimumab Works:

Belimumab is designed to inhibit the activity of B-lymphocyte stimulator (BLyS) protein. BLyS is crucial for the survival and differentiation of B cells, a type of white blood cell involved in the immune response. By targeting BLyS, belimumab reduces the proliferation of B cells. However, in lupus and lupus nephritis, B cells are activated, but there are other immune cells that are activated. Hence, Belimumab should be used in conjunction with MMF rather than alone by itself for the treatment of lupus nephritis.

Advantages of Belimumab:

The advantage of belimumab is that it targets a specific pathway that causes inflammation in patients with lupus nephritis. As discussed above, using belimumab along with MMF is a combination therapy that helps target specific inflammatory pathways and, hence, individualized treatment plans for patients with lupus nephritis. When Belimumab was used with MMF, more patients with lupus nephritis went into remission despite a lower dose of corticosteroids. This decreased the side effects of corticosteroids, such as weight gain, diabetes, bone disease, cataracts, etc. Belimumab works especially well to decrease the inflammation in joints and skin along with kidneys and, hence a good medication for someone with symptoms like joint pain and swelling along with lupus nephritis. Hence, combination therapy for lupus nephritis of MMF with belimumab should be considered for someone with lupus nephritis and significant systemic symptoms for lupus. This personalization of an immunosuppressant treatment plan is the future for lupus nephritis with the aim of effectively controlling the disease and decreasing inflammation in the kidneys to preserve kidney function along with minimizing the side effects of the medications.

Side effects of Belimumab:

Belimumab is an immunosuppressant and hence associated with a higher risk of infections. It is a new drug and, hence, significantly expensive compared to other medications. Belimumab is given intravenously and hence requires a visit to the infusion center every 2-4 weeks. There is a subcutaneous self-injector available that patients can use to inject themselves at home, however, that formulation has not been studied for the treatment of lupus nephritis.

F. Anti-CD 20 monoclonal antibody: Rituximab and Obinutuzumab

Rituximab and Obinutuzumab are monoclonal antibodies specifically designed to target CD20, a protein found on the surface of B cells. Both these medications specifically kill B cells in the body and target only this cell population. They are different in how they kill B cells in the body. Rituximab is an older medication and has been studied in lupus nephritis. It plays a crucial role in cases where patients do not respond adequately to conventional treatments (30-33). Obinutuzumab was recently studied for the treatment of lupus nephritis along with MMF and has been shown to increase the risk of complete remission along with the use of lower doses of corticosteroids. It is not yet FDA-approved for lupus nephritis but likely will get approved for treatment of lupus nephritis this year, given the positive studies in patients with lupus nephritis.

How Obinutuzumab and Rituximab Works:

Both Obinutuzumab and Rituximab work by binding to the CD20 molecule on B cells, a type of white blood cell involved in the immune response. By binding to these cells, Obinutuzumab and Rituximab mark them for destruction by the body's immune system. This process effectively reduces the number of B cells that produce antibodies that can attack the body's tissues in autoimmune diseases like lupus.

Application in Lupus Nephritis:

In lupus nephritis, where the immune system attacks the kidneys, causing inflammation and damage, the reduction in the B cell population can decrease the severity of the autoimmune attack on kidney tissues.

Safety and Side Effects:

1. Infusion Reactions: Rituximab and Obinutuzumab are administered via infusion, and patients can experience reactions such as fever, chills, and nausea during or shortly after the injection. This is easily manageable with medications like Tylenol, Benadryl, and corticosteroids with the infusion.

2. Infection Risk: As with other immunosuppressants, there is an increased risk of infections, given the critical role of B cells in the immune defense system.

Long-term Safety:

Ongoing research is needed to understand the long-term safety of rituximab and obinutuzumab in lupus nephritis, especially regarding potential impacts on immune function.

Obinutuzumab has been studied in randomized controlled trials and is an effective treatment of Lupus Nephritis. However, the long-term effects of Obinutuzumab have not been studied as the studies are recent. Rituximab offers an off-label option for treating lupus nephritis, particularly in patients who have not responded to other therapies. Its targeted approach provides a focused method to combat the underlying autoimmune mechanisms of the disease.

G. Azathioprine:

Azathioprine is a medication used for maintenance therapy for lupus nephritis. The maintenance therapy is used to prevent the relapse of lupus nephritis after treatment of lupus nephritis (34-36). The significant advantage of azathioprine is that it is one of the safest immunosuppressant medications that can be used in pregnancy to treat lupus nephritis. It is also used in patients that cannot tolerate or are allergic to mycophenolate

How Azathioprine Works:

Azathioprine inhibits the proliferation of specific white blood cells responsible for the autoimmune response in lupus nephritis. By curbing the growth of these cells, azathioprine helps reduce the overall immune response, thereby preventing the immune system from attacking the kidney tissues. This action helps extend the remission periods and control the disease with a lower burden of side effects.

Side effects:

Azathioprine is an immunosuppressant and can lead to an increased risk of infections. Azathioprine can lead to bone marrow suppression, low white blood cell count, anemia, and platelet cell count. Thus, patients on azathioprine need to have their blood tests monitored regularly.

 # Non-Immunosuppressants:

Non-immunosuppressive medications are also used to treat lupus nephritis, primarily to manage symptoms and prevent complications.

A. Antimalarial Drugs:

Hydroxychloroquine is a widely used medication in managing lupus, including lupus nephritis. Its role extends beyond simply treating the symptoms; it helps reduce the frequency of disease flares and provides a protective effect against the progression of lupus into the kidneys (37, 38).

Mechanism of Action:

Hydroxychloroquine belongs to a class of drugs known as antimalarials, but its benefits in lupus are due to its anti-inflammatory and immunomodulatory properties. It works by inhibiting specific cellular processes involved in the immune response. Doing so reduces inflammation and helps calm the overactive immune system that characterizes lupus.

Benefits in Lupus and Lupus Nephritis Treatment:

1. Reduction of Flares: Regular hydroxychloroquine has significantly reduced the number of flares in lupus patients. This is crucial as each flare can lead to increased tissue damage, including the kidneys (39, 40).

2. Prevention of Organ Damage: By controlling disease activity, hydroxychloroquine helps prevent or slow the progression of damage to vital organs, including the kidneys. Its use is associated with a lower risk of developing lupus nephritis, one of the more serious complications of systemic lupus erythematosus (41).

3. Long-Term Benefits: Studies have suggested that lupus patients taking hydroxychloroquine over long periods have better overall outcomes, including reduced cumulative damage and improved survival rates (41).

Managing Side Effects:

Hydroxychloroquine is generally well-tolerated by most patients, making it suitable for long-term use. However, it can have some side effects, such as:

1. Eye Toxicity: One of the more serious concerns with hydroxychloroquine is the potential for retinal damage, which can lead to vision problems. Regular eye exams are recommended for patients using the drug for extended periods to catch any signs of toxicity early.

2. Gastrointestinal Issues: Some patients may experience stomach cramps, nausea, or diarrhea, although these symptoms are usually mild and can often be managed with adjustments to the dosage or timing of medication.

3. Skin Reactions: Although rare, hydroxychloroquine can cause skin rashes or itchiness, which usually resolves after discontinuing the drug.

Hydroxychloroquine is a cornerstone in managing lupus because it reduces flare-ups and protects against kidney damage. Its immunomodulatory effects make it invaluable, particularly in preventing the progression of lupus nephritis. With careful monitoring, particularly for eye health, hydroxychloroquine is a critical tool in long-term lupus management, offering patients a better quality of life and improved disease outcomes.

B. ACE Inhibitors and ARBs:

In managing lupus nephritis, one of the goals is to decrease the protein in the urine. ACE-I/ARB helps reduce protein in the urine. ACE-I/ARB also controls high blood pressure, crucial to preserving kidney health and function. High blood pressure is not only a common symptom of kidney disease but also a significant risk factor that can accelerate the progression of kidney damage (42-44).

Role of ACE-I and ARBs:

1. Reducing Proteinuria:

Mechanism: ACE- I and ARBs are particularly effective in reducing proteinuria. They lower the pressure inside the glomeruli (kidney filtering units), which decreases the amount of protein that leaks into the urine.

Impact: Reducing proteinuria is beneficial because excessive protein in the urine can be a sign of kidney damage. High protein in the urine causes further damage to the kidneys. By controlling proteinuria, these medications help protect kidney function and can slow the progression of kidney disease.

2. Lowering Blood Pressure:

Mechanism: ACE I/ARB works by inhibiting the production of angiotensin II, a substance in the body that narrows blood vessels. By preventing the formation of angiotensin II, these drugs help relax and dilate blood vessels, which lowers blood pressure. ARBs, on the other hand, block angiotensin II from binding to its receptors. This also helps relax blood vessels and reduces blood pressure.

Impact: Lowering blood pressure in patients with lupus nephritis is vital as it helps reduce the strain on the kidneys, slowing the progression of kidney damage and reducing the risk of cardiovascular complications.

Benefits and Considerations:

Cardiovascular Benefits: Besides their effects on the kidneys, ACE-I and ARBs have cardiovascular benefits, which are essential given the increased risk of heart disease in patients with chronic kidney disease and lupus.

Side Effects: While generally safe and well-tolerated, these medications can have side effects such as cough (more common with ACE-I), elevated potassium levels, fatigue, and dizziness. ACE-I/ARB is also contraindicated in pregnancy due to potential harm to the developing fetus.

Monitoring Requirements: Regular monitoring of kidney function and potassium levels is necessary when using these medications, especially since lupus nephritis can affect kidney function.

ACE-I and ARBs in lupus nephritis address two crucial aspects of the disease—high blood pressure and proteinuria—vital to preventing further kidney damage and maintaining overall kidney health. Their role in reducing the risk of cardiovascular disease adds a layer of benefit, making them integral components of the management strategy for lupus nephritis. Their effectiveness underscores the importance of comprehensive care in treating this complex autoimmune disease.

C. Diuretics:

Diuretics, commonly referred to as water pills, are frequently prescribed to patients with lupus nephritis to help manage symptoms of fluid retention and swelling. These medications are essential in controlling excess fluid buildup in the body, a common issue when the kidneys are not functioning properly due to lupus nephritis.

How Diuretics Work:

Diuretics influence the kidneys' ability to regulate water and salt balance. They promote the excretion of water and sodium through urine. This action helps normalize the volume of fluid circulating through the blood vessels, as lupus nephritis causes the kidneys to retain more salt and water, causing an imbalance in salt and water homeostasis.

Types of Diuretics:

There are different types of diuretics, and each works in a slightly different way:

1. Thiazide Diuretics (Hydrochlorothiazide): Thiazide diuretics are often recommended to help with mild to moderate swelling and high blood pressure by aiding the body in getting rid of extra salt and water through urine. These medications can effectively lower blood pressure and alleviate swelling by reducing the body's water content, mainly by flushing out excess salt. One possible side effect of thiazide diuretics is the loss of potassium, an essential mineral for muscle and heart health, which might cause weakness or cramps. To help counteract this, healthcare providers may suggest incorporating potassium-rich foods into your diet or taking supplements.

2. Loop Diuretics (Furosemide): Loop diuretics are strong medications that are helpful when removing excess fluid quickly, especially in serious cases of swelling related to heart or kidney issues. These diuretics work on the loop of Henle in the kidneys, which helps control how much water the body keeps. Promoting the release of salt, potassium, and water leads to more frequent urination, effectively reducing swelling and fluid buildup in no time. However, one possible side effect of loop diuretics is the depletion of essential minerals like potassium, calcium, and magnesium, which can cause muscle cramps or impact heart health. To avoid these issues, healthcare providers carefully monitor blood mineral levels.

3. Potassium-Sparing Diuretics (Spironolactone): Potassium-sparing diuretics are unique in that they help the body eliminate excess water while preserving potassium levels. These diuretics are often used alongside other diuretics to maintain a balance of minerals in the body. They block a hormone called aldosterone, which typically causes the body to retain salt and water. By blocking this hormone, potassium-sparing diuretics help remove excess water without depleting potassium. A critical side effect is the risk of elevated potassium levels, which can threaten heart function. To mitigate this risk, healthcare providers regularly monitor potassium levels to ensure they remain within a safe range.

Benefits of Diuretics in Lupus Nephritis:

In lupus nephritis, fluid buildup in the body can cause swelling in the legs, ankles, feet, abdomen, and around the eyes. Diuretics can help manage this condition by removing excess fluid from the body.

One benefit of diuretics is that they reduce swelling, which helps ease discomfort. Diuretics help relieve the pressure that causes the swelling by making the body release extra fluid.

Another advantage is that diuretics can improve breathing. In cases where fluid builds up in or around the lungs, diuretics help reduce this fluid, making breathing easier.

Diuretics can also help lower blood pressure. By decreasing the amount of fluid in the blood vessels, diuretics help to lower blood pressure, which is beneficial for kidney health, especially in people with lupus nephritis.

Considerations and Side Effects:

Diuretics are effective for managing fluid retention in conditions like lupus nephritis, but they must be used with caution due to potential side effects. These medications help the kidneys remove excess water and salt but can lead to imbalances in essential electrolytes, dehydration, kidney strain, and low blood pressure. Here are the main concerns and ways to manage them:

1. Electrolyte Imbalance: Diuretics can cause the body to lose important electrolytes like potassium, sodium, and magnesium. Potassium loss can cause muscle cramps, weakness, and abnormal heart rhythms. Potassium supplements or potassium-rich foods like bananas and spinach may be recommended to manage this. Regular blood tests and hydration are essential for sodium and magnesium imbalances, with supplements given as needed.

2. Dehydration: By increasing water excretion, diuretics can lead to dehydration if not properly managed. Symptoms like dry mouth, dizziness, and dark-colored urine may occur, and severe dehydration can cause low blood pressure or kidney damage. To prevent this, it's important to drink plenty of fluids, especially when starting diuretics, and regularly monitor fluid levels with medical providers.

3. Impact on Kidney Function: Diuretics can stress the kidneys, especially in people with lupus nephritis. This can worsen kidney function or increase blood creatinine levels, signaling kidney strain. Regular monitoring of kidney function is necessary, and adjustments to the diuretic dose may be made to protect the kidneys.

4. Low Blood Pressure (Hypotension): Diuretics can sometimes lower blood pressure too much, causing dizziness or fainting, especially when standing. To manage this, doctors may adjust the dosage or timing of diuretics, and it's helpful for patients to stand up slowly to avoid dizziness.

Although diuretics are essential in treating symptoms of lupus nephritis, especially fluid buildup, careful monitoring and adjustments are necessary to prevent complications and ensure the treatment's effectiveness.

Conclusion

Treating lupus nephritis is a journey that requires both strength and patience. The induction and maintenance phases may seem demanding, but they are carefully designed to control inflammation, protect your kidneys, and give you the best chance at long-term health. While the medications can have side effects, your healthcare team will work closely with you to manage them and adjust treatment as needed.

The most important message is this: you are not powerless. With modern therapies, supportive care, and a personalized plan, many people with lupus nephritis achieve remission and return to living full, meaningful lives. Every step — from taking your medicines to regular check-ups — brings you closer to protecting your kidneys and building a future filled with hope.

Take home points

- Lupus nephritis treatment involves an induction phase to control inflammation and a maintenance phase to sustain remission and prevent relapse.
- Immunosuppressants are essential for treating lupus nephritis to prevent damage to the kidneys but require close monitoring due to potential side effects like infections.
- Long-term corticosteroid use can lead to side effects such as weight gain and bone loss.
- Diuretics help manage fluid retention but must be used cautiously to avoid dehydration and electrolyte imbalances.
- A newer treatment regimen for lupus nephritis focuses on low-dose corticosteroids and a combination of two immunosuppressants to attain faster disease remission to prevent ongoing damage to the kidneys

References

1. Mok CC. Understanding lupus nephritis: diagnosis, management, and treatment options. Int J Womens Health. 2012;4:213-22.
2. Mejia-Vilet JM, Ayoub I. The Use of Glucocorticoids in Lupus Nephritis: New Pathways for an Old Drug. Front Med (Lausanne). 2021;8:622225.
3. Chan TM. Lupus nephritis: induction therapy. Lupus. 2005;14 Suppl 1:s27-32.
4. Ponticelli C, Glassock RJ, Moroni G. Induction and maintenance therapy in proliferative lupus nephritis. J Nephrol. 2010;23(1):9-16.
5. Buchman AL. Side effects of corticosteroid therapy. J Clin Gastroenterol. 2001;33(4):289-94.
6. Yasir M, Goyal A, Sonthalia S. Corticosteroid Adverse Effects. StatPearls. Treasure Island (FL)2024.
7. Oray M, Abu Samra K, Ebrahimiadib N, Meese H, Foster CS. Long-term side effects of glucocorticoids. Expert Opin Drug Saf. 2016;15(4):457-65.
8. Koshi EJ, Young K, Mostales JC, Vo KB, Burgess LP. Complications of Corticosteroid Therapy: A Comprehensive Literature Review. J Pharm Technol. 2022;38(6):360-7.

9. Struck RF, Alberts DS, Horne K, Phillips JG, Peng YM, Roe DJ. Plasma pharmacokinetics of cyclophosphamide and its cytotoxic metabolites after intravenous versus oral administration in a randomized, crossover trial. Cancer Res. 1987;47(10):2723-6.
10. Donadio JV, Jr., Holley KE, Ferguson RH, Ilstrup DM. Treatment of diffuse proliferative lupus nephritis with prednisone and combined prednisone and cyclophosphamide. N Engl J Med. 1978;299(21):1151-5.
11. Gourley MF, Austin HA, 3rd, Scott D, Yarboro CH, Vaughan EM, Muir J, et al. Methylprednisolone and cyclophosphamide, alone or in combination, in patients with lupus nephritis. A randomized, controlled trial. Ann Intern Med. 1996;125(7):549-57.
12. Ahmed AR, Hombal SM. Cyclophosphamide (Cytoxan). A review on relevant pharmacology and clinical uses. J Am Acad Dermatol. 1984;11(6):1115-26.
13. Ogino MH, Tadi P. Cyclophosphamide. StatPearls. Treasure Island (FL)2024.
14. Fraiser LH, Kanekal S, Kehrer JP. Cyclophosphamide toxicity. Characterising and avoiding the problem. Drugs. 1991;42(5):781-95.
15. Martin F, Lauwerys B, Lefebvre C, Devogelaer JP, Houssiau FA. Side-effects of intravenous cyclophosphamide pulse therapy. Lupus. 1997;6(3):254-7.
16. Hahn BH, McMahon MA, Wilkinson A, Wallace WD, Daikh DI, Fitzgerald JD, et al. American College of Rheumatology guidelines for screening, treatment, and management of lupus nephritis. Arthritis Care Res (Hoboken). 2012;64(6):797-808.
17. Bertsias GK, Tektonidou M, Amoura Z, Aringer M, Bajema I, Berden JH, et al. Joint European League Against Rheumatism and European Renal Association-European Dialysis and Transplant Association (EULAR/ERA-EDTA) recommendations for the management of adult and paediatric lupus nephritis. Ann Rheum Dis. 2012;71(11):1771-82.
18. Appel AS, Appel GB. An update on the use of mycophenolate mofetil in lupus nephritis and other primary glomerular diseases. Nat Clin Pract Nephrol. 2009;5(3):132-42.
19. Appel GB, Contreras G, Dooley MA, Ginzler EM, Isenberg D, Jayne D, et al. Mycophenolate mofetil versus cyclophosphamide for induction treatment of lupus nephritis. J Am Soc Nephrol. 2009;20(5):1103-12.
20. Radhakrishnan J, Moutzouris DA, Ginzler EM, Solomons N, Siempos, II, Appel GB. Mycophenolate mofetil and intravenous

cyclophosphamide are similar as induction therapy for class V lupus nephritis. Kidney Int. 2010;77(2):152-60.
21. Aziz F, Chaudhary K. Lupus Nephritis: A Treatment Update. Curr Clin Pharmacol. 2018;13(1):4-13.
22. Behrend M. Adverse gastrointestinal effects of mycophenolate mofetil: aetiology, incidence and management. Drug Saf. 2001; 24(9):645-63.
23. Kamanamool N, McEvoy M, Attia J, Ingsathit A, Ngamjanyaporn P, Thakkinstian A. Efficacy and adverse events of mycophenolate mofetil versus cyclophosphamide for induction therapy of lupus nephritis: systematic review and meta-analysis. Medicine (Baltimore). 2010;89(4):227-35.
24. Bunnapradist S, Ambuhl PM. Impact of gastrointestinal-related side effects on mycophenolate mofetil dosing and potential therapeutic strategies. Clin Transplant. 2008;22(6):815-21.
25. Sobiak J, Kaminska J, Glyda M, Duda G, Chrzanowska M. Effect of mycophenolate mofetil on hematological side effects incidence in renal transplant recipients. Clin Transplant. 2013;27(4):E407-14.
26. Siepmann K, Huber M, Stubiger N, Deuter C, Zierhut M. Mycophenolate mofetil is a highly effective and safe immunosuppressive agent for the treatment of uveitis : a retrospective analysis of 106 patients. Graefes Arch Clin Exp Ophthalmol. 2006;244(7):788-94.
27. Kirou KA, Salmon JE, Crow MK. Soluble mediators as therapeutic targets in systemic lupus erythematosus: cytokines, immunoglobulin receptors, and the complement system. Rheum Dis Clin North Am. 2006;32(1):103-19, ix.
28. Manzi S, Sanchez-Guerrero J, Merrill JT, Furie R, Gladman D, Navarra SV, et al. Effects of belimumab, a B lymphocyte stimulator-specific inhibitor, on disease activity across multiple organ domains in patients with systemic lupus erythematosus: combined results from two phase III trials. Ann Rheum Dis. 2012;71(11):1833-8.
29. De Scheerder MA, Boey O, Mahieu E, Vanuytsel J, Bogaert AM. Case report: successful treatment of membranous lupus nephritis with belimumab in an African female immigrant. Clin Rheumatol. 2016;35(6):1649-53.
30. Rovin BH, Furie R, Latinis K, Looney RJ, Fervenza FC, Sanchez-Guerrero J, et al. Efficacy and safety of rituximab in patients with active proliferative lupus nephritis: the Lupus Nephritis Assessment with Rituximab study. Arthritis Rheum. 2012;64(4):1215-26.

31. Camous L, Melander C, Vallet M, Squalli T, Knebelmann B, Noel LH, et al. Complete remission of lupus nephritis with rituximab and steroids for induction and rituximab alone for maintenance therapy. Am J Kidney Dis. 2008;52(2):346-52.
32. Fra GP, Avanzi GC, Bartoli E. Remission of refractory lupus nephritis with a protocol including rituximab. Lupus. 2003;12(10): 783-7.
33. Vigna-Perez M, Hernandez-Castro B, Paredes-Saharopulos O, Portales-Perez D, Baranda L, Abud-Mendoza C, et al. Clinical and immunological effects of Rituximab in patients with lupus nephritis refractory to conventional therapy: a pilot study. Arthritis Res Ther. 2006;8(3):R83.
34. Grootscholten C, Ligtenberg G, Hagen EC, van den Wall Bake AW, de Glas-Vos JW, Bijl M, et al. Azathioprine/methylprednisolone versus cyclophosphamide in proliferative lupus nephritis. A randomized controlled trial. Kidney Int. 2006;70(4):732-42.
35. Feldman CH, Collins J, Zhang Z, Xu C, Subramanian SV, Kawachi I, et al. Azathioprine and Mycophenolate Mofetil Adherence Patterns and Predictors Among Medicaid Beneficiaries With Systemic Lupus Erythematosus. Arthritis Care Res (Hoboken). 2019;71(11):1419-24.
36. Nossent HC, Koldingsnes W. Long-term efficacy of azathioprine treatment for proliferative lupus nephritis. Rheumatology (Oxford). 2000;39(9):969-74.
37. Gheet FS, Dawoud HE, El-Shahaby WA, Elrifaey SM, Abdelnabi HH. Hydroxychloroquine in children with proliferative lupus nephritis: a randomized clinical trial. Eur J Pediatr. 2023;182(4): 1685-95.
38. Dima A, Jurcut C, Chasset F, Felten R, Arnaud L. Hydroxychloroquine in systemic lupus erythematosus: overview of current knowledge. Ther Adv Musculoskelet Dis. 2022;14:1759720X211073001.
39. Kasitanon N, Fine DM, Haas M, Magder LS, Petri M. Hydroxychloroquine use predicts complete renal remission within 12 months among patients treated with mycophenolate mofetil therapy for membranous lupus nephritis. Lupus. 2006;15(6):366-70.
40. Mejia-Vilet JM, Cordova-Sanchez BM, Uribe-Uribe NO, Correa-Rotter R. Immunosuppressive treatment for pure membranous lupus nephropathy in a Hispanic population. Clin Rheumatol. 2016;35(9): 2219-27.
41. Pena-Vizcarra OR, Zavala-Miranda MF, Juarez-Cuevas B, Marquez-Macedo SE, Hernandez-Andrade A, Nordmann-Gomes A,

et al. Effect of antimalarials on clinical outcomes in lupus nephritis. Rheumatology (Oxford). 2024;63(8):2230-8.
42. Tse KC, Li FK, Tang S, Tang CS, Lai KN, Chan TM. Angiotensin inhibition or blockade for the treatment of patients with quiescent lupus nephritis and persistent proteinuria. Lupus. 2005;14(12):947-52.
43. De Albuquerque DA, Saxena V, Adams DE, Boivin GP, Brunner HI, Witte DP, et al. An ACE inhibitor reduces Th2 cytokines and TGF-beta1 and TGF-beta2 isoforms in murine lupus nephritis. Kidney Int. 2004;65(3):846-59.
44. Duran-Barragan S, McGwin G, Jr., Vila LM, Reveille JD, Alarcon GS, cohort LamU. Angiotensin-converting enzyme inhibitors delay the occurrence of renal involvement and are associated with a decreased risk of disease activity in patients with systemic lupus erythematosus--results from LUMINA (LIX): a multiethnic US cohort. Rheumatology (Oxford). 2008;47(7):1093-6.

CHAPTER 6

YOUR GUIDE TO MEDICATIONS

SIMPLE STEPS TO STAY ON TRACK WITH TREATMENT

BY SHIVANI GARG MD PHD

ASSOCIATE PROFESSOR, DIVISION OF RHEUMATOLOGY, DEPARTMENT OF MEDICINE

MEDICAL DIRECTOR OF UNIVERSITY OF WISCONSIN'S LUPUS AND LUPUS NEPHRITIS CLINICS

UNIVERSITY OF WISCONSIN, SCHOOL OF MEDICINE AND PUBLIC HEALTH, MADISON

Abstract

Living with lupus nephritis often means managing a daily routine of multiple medicines, which can feel overwhelming. This chapter provides practical guidance to help patients stay consistent with their treatments and understand why medicines are so important. Through a hypothetical story, it highlights the emotional challenges of medication routines while offering reassurance that medicines act as shields, protecting the kidneys and preventing long-term damage. Readers will learn simple strategies — such as pill organizers, phone reminders, discussing side effects, and seeking financial assistance — to make adherence easier. The chapter also emphasizes the importance of regular blood and urine tests, personalized dosing, and building a strong partnership with the healthcare team. By understanding and embracing their medicines, patients can take control of lupus nephritis, reduce flares, safeguard their kidneys, and live healthier, fuller lives.

Keywords: Lupus Nephritis, Medications, Adherence, Side Effects, Kidney Protection.

Let's start the chapter with the hypothetical story of Maria. Maria sat at her kitchen table, staring at the little row of pill bottles lined neatly by the coffee pot. It had only been three months since her diagnosis, and already the daily routine of medicines felt overwhelming. Some mornings she forgot a dose. Other mornings she debated whether the side effects — the nausea, the bloating — were worth it.

She sighed, remembering the weeks before treatment: the swelling in her ankles, the crushing fatigue that made climbing stairs feel impossible, and the fear of what her kidneys were silently going through. Those memories steadied her hand as she reached for her pillbox.

Maria reminded herself that these medicines weren't punishments; they were shields. Each pill worked quietly to protect her kidneys, reduce inflammation, and keep her moving forward. They gave her strength to return to her job, laugh with her children, and plan for the future.

As she swallowed the tablets with her morning coffee, Maria whispered to herself, *"I have lupus, but lupus doesn't have me."* And with that, she stepped into her day — a little stronger, a little more in control.

Like Maria, many people with lupus nephritis find taking medicines challenging, but with the right tools and strategies, medicines can become trusted allies in the journey toward health.

Living with lupus and lupus nephritis can feel like a full-time job. On top of everything else, trying to keep track of medicines every day could be difficult, particularly when medicines need to be taken for months, sometimes years or decades. However, when you feel that you are struggling, try to remember this powerful idea: **"I have lupus, lupus doesn't have me."** You are in the driver's seat of your health journey. Additionally, medicines are your friends as they will help you stay in the driver's seat and make the journey smooth and easy.

Everyday waking up to take medicines, can be a real challenge. Moreover, trying to understand how medicines work, what to look out for in terms of side effects, alternative medicines, medical bills and co-pays, and how to balance side effects with daily functioning, can further add complexities in decision-making around lupus medicines. We have prepared this guide to give you simple, practical tips to make taking your medicines easier, so that you can focus on living your life to the fullest potential. Additionally, it will help you partner with your healthcare team to identify alternative medicines, different formulations with less side effects, or coupons to lower drug costs.

The most important thing to remember is that your medicines are your friends. They can be hard sometimes but will help you and your health in the long run. As you may know, lupus affects your immune system where your immune system can get confused and attack healthy parts of your body, including your skin, joints, kidneys (this is called lupus nephritis), heart, lungs, and even brain.[1-12] Lupus attack can sometimes be silent, particularly when it affects kidneys as you may not have many symptoms early during lupus nephritis disease course. If the inflammation in the kidney remains unchecked or uncontrolled, it can scar your organs and cause irreversible damage.[5,13-17] Therefore, it is very important to control the inflammation.

The medicines that you take for lupus decrease the inflammation in your body and organs like kidney. Think about lupus medicines as your defenders against the inflammation due to lupus; they work 24/7 to calm your immune system down and protect your organs. However, these medicines work 24/7, only when taken regularly. The medicines are not just when your get symptoms from lupus and lupus nephritis.

Common medicines for lupus control include hydroxychloroquine (Plaquenil), mycophenolate (CellCept), Azathioprine (Imuran), Benlysta, Tacrolimus, Lupkynis etc. Among these medicines, hydroxychloroquine (Plaquenil) treats lupus and lupus nephritis but also prevents more flares of lupus and lupus nephritis.[18-29] Likewise, other medicines can further calm down the inflammation in your body.

Taking medicines regularly can help you take control back over your lupus, as they will:

- **Prevent Flares:** Keep lupus from suddenly getting worse.
- **Protect Your Kidneys:** Stop or slow down damage to your kidneys.
- **Reduce Long-Term Damage:** Protect your organs over many years.
- **Prolong Your Life:** Increases chances of survival.

So, every day when you take your medicines, think of them as a shield. For the shield to work best, you must hold it up every day.

Here are some simple tips for taking your medicines regularly.

It is completely normal to forget a dose—especially when you feel tired or are dealing with "lupus fog" and life. The key is to have a system that works for you, so you don't have to rely only on memory.

Here a Few Tips that might work for You:

Tips	How it helps
Make it a Habit	Link taking your pills to something you already do every day, like making your morning coffee, getting ready for bed, brushing your teeth, or having a meal
Pillbox	A weekly pill organizer is a tool to keep a track of medicines you have taken or forgotten during the week
Phone Alarms	Use your phone's alarm or a free medication reminder app to give you a nudge
Discuss Side Effects	Are you worried about how a medicine makes you feel? Don't just stop taking it. Discuss with your doctor and healthcare team. They can often help you manage side effects or find a different medicine that works better for you
Alternative Choices	There are alternative choices for medications that can reduce side effects. For example, Mycophenolate aka Cellcept comes in two formulations, mycophenolic acid and Myfortic. For some people mycophenolic acid is better tolerated and myfortic for others. A simple switch could help you tolerate this life saving medicine better while living your life on your terms
Ask Your Doctors to Discuss Benefits vs. Harms of the Medicines	Knowing more about the medicines or having better understanding of how long the medicine can take to work and the side effects, can help you align your expectations to medicine response better. Additionally, it can help you be prepared for a bad day or a side effect. Studies have shown that knowing more about significant benefits vs. low harms of taking medicines like Hydroxychloroquine (Plaquenil) supported patients in navigating complex treatment decisions and feel more confident about taking the medicine.[31,32] So, ask your doctor if they can review such shared decision-making educational tool, like hcqsafe.medicine.wisc.edu, with you

Partner with a Pharmacist	Pharmacists can help you understand your medicines better. They can walk you through the benefits of taking the medicine and guide to limit side effects. They can work with your doctor and insurance companies to decrease the cost of medications
Ask about Co-pay Assistance or Coupons	Medicines can be costly. Discuss with your healthcare team including your doctor and/or pharmacist. There are drug coupons or co-pay assistance that can be used to offset some of the cost of the medicines. Websites like GoodRx.com, costplusdrugs.com, are good resources to look for more affordable medicine prices
Enroll in mail-order pharmacy and get medicines delivered at your doorstep	If you have been having trouble getting medicines refills on time because the pharmacy had closed by the time you wrapped up work, or picked up your kids, mail-order pharmacy is the right choice for you. Several insurance companies cover the costs of delivering medicines at your doorstep. Ask your healthcare team or pharmacist today how you can enroll in such services.
Talk to a Friend or Family Member	Often discussing with a friend in similar situation, or a family member can help you share your fears and plan better. You can even connect with other patients living with lupus like yourself by joining a support group. You can find lupus support groups online, or by navigating lupus.org, an official site of the Lupus Foundation of America

Blood and urine tests are needed to monitor treatment response

Blood and urine tests often can serve as a report card for your kidneys and lupus control. Therefore, regular blood and urine tests are extremely important. They show how well your medicines are protecting your kidneys. Getting your labs done on time helps your doctor make sure your treatment plan is working well. It is recommend to get blood and urine tests done, particularly if you have lupus nephritis, every 3-6 months.[34,35] This frequency can be changed based on your lupus activity, therefore, it is important to develop a care and lab monitoring plan with your healthcare team that works for you and your lupus.

Additionally, there are new blood tests that can check the level of medicines that is getting absorbed in your blood. This information will help you and your doctor understand if the dose that you are taking is safe for you and working for you. Often it is referred as a therapeutic range or **the "Safe Zone" or "sweet spot."[36]** Blood levels are routinely measured for **Prograf aka Tacrolimus** to ensure that the dose is not too high risking side effects. At the same time, Tacrolimus blood levels also guide if the dose is not low that could risk lupus flares.

By doing so, the dose of Tacrolimus or Prograf can be tailored to a person's absorption and metabolism rather than giving everyone the same dose (often called as "one-size-fits-all" doses). Likewise, there is growing evidence on **measuring hydroxychloroquine (Plaquenil) blood levels** to identify the "sweet spot" or a "protection zone" for this medicine in your blood.[36-55] When your level is in this zone, you have a much lower chance of having a lupus flare. Additionally, knowing blood hydroxychloroquine levels also prevents side effects from very high blood levels. Therefore, monitoring these levels ensures that the dose is safe and effective. Additionally, monitoring **mycophenolate levels** can also help reduce the dose to limit stomach related side effects, particularly in children and certain ethnic groups. More importantly, testing for most of these medicine levels are now covered by insurance companies.

Overall, measuring medicine levels in blood could help your doctor tailor your medicine's dose based on your body's absorption and metabolism. Taking a tailored or personalized dosing regimen for life-saving medicines could be the best way to bring balance in using lupus nephritis medicines with least side effects. Ask your doctor if/how you can get a medicine blood level monitoring done.

Cost of medications

The medications for treatment of lupus and lupus nephritis can be very expensive even with insurance coverage. But that should not add to your worry and affect your medicine regimen or treatment plan. Know that you always have options!

Here a few resources and tips for you:

- **Always Ask for Generics:** Always ask your doctor if there is a generic version of your medicine. They have the same exact medicine in them but usually cost much less.
- **Try New Online Pharmacies:** Check out websites that offer low-cost medicines. A great example is the **Mark Cuban Cost Plus Drug Company**: Prices for chronic medicines, like mycophenolate, hydroxychloroquine, are very reasonable. Your doctor can send the prescription to these online pharmacies directly and the medicines are delivered to your house! Other options: Amazon, Walmart offers such services as well.
- **Use Coupon Websites:** Websites like **GoodRx** offer free coupons you can use at almost any pharmacy to lower the price.
- **Ask Your Doctor's Office for Help:** Your doctor, pharmacist, nurse, or social worker may know about special programs from drug companies that help patients pay for their medicine. Do not hesitate to ask.
- **Apply for Health Grants:** Organizations like Lupus Foundation of America, HealthWell Foundation, Patient Advocate Foundation, etc. offer health or medial grants that can cover medical bills or medicine costs. You might have to complete an application form and show financial documentation to get approved. There is a chance not everyone is eligible for these grants so discuss with your pharmacist or local health advocate about these resources and eligibility criteria.
- **Apply to Pharmaceutical Companies to Get Your Co-Pay Assistance Cards:** You might be eligible to get a co-pay assistance card through a pharmaceutical company to cover costs of medicines like mycophenolic acid, belimumab or voclosporin. If you are on such medicines, then ask your healthcare team today about the process to apply for these co-pay assistance cards.

Finally, remember that you and your healthcare team are in this together. Therefore, having a strong rapport and a relationship aka a powerful partnership with your healthcare team is important.[56,57] As an expert in lupus and treating people living with lupus for more than a decade, I have learnt the managing lupus is a team sport, and you (patient) are the captain of the team. When choosing your team members, make sure you include a rheumatologist whom you trust, a kidney doctor aka nephrologist if you have kidney lupus, a pharmacist, a primary care doctor. This team might be bigger and include a skin doctor aka dermatologist, lung doctor aka pulmonologist or a heart doctor or a cardiologist based on your symptoms. However, the most important thing is that you should build a team that you trust and who know you and your lupus inside out! Moreover, make sure that your team is aware of all updates and your team talk to each other so that you get the best care that you deserve.

Here a Few Things to Consider When You are Preparing to Meet Your Doctor:

- **Be Open and Honest:** Your doctors should/will never judge you. If you're having trouble, tell them. You can say, "I've been finding it hard to remember my pills in the morning because of brain fog or I have to rush to get to work. Do you have any suggestions?" or "I'm worried about the side effects of this medicine."
- **Write It Down:** Before your visit, write down your questions. It's easy to forget things once you're in the office.
- **Take a Family Member or Friend to a Clinic Visit:** It might be a good idea to take a family member or a friend to a clinic visit so that they can advocate for you and understand what you are going through. This will feel emotionally supported through this journey.
- **Ask for a Clear Medicine Regimen or Care Plan:** At the end of your visit, ask for a simple, written summary of your plan. Also, ask if this plan can be shared with you and other members on your healthcare team.
- **Are You Feeling Depressed:** Lupus is a chronic disease and can be challenging and often depressing. Know that there is light at the end of this tunnel, and the only way to find out is to keep moving forward. If you are experiencing depression or mood changes, call your doctor today!
- **Some Medicines and Viruses can be Harmful:** Ask your doctor or pharmacist if some medicines like an antibiotic (Bactrim) is right for you, as it can trigger a lupus and lupus nephritis flare. Likewise, viruses can trigger mild to severe lupus flare, so taking vaccinations could prevent such infections. However, consult your doctor before taking vaccines.
- **Celebrate Your Wins:** When your lab tests look good, take a moment to be proud. It's proof that all your hard work is paying off!
- **Ups and Downs:** Lupus Nephritis can flare. Remember, experiencing a flare is a common part of living with lupus and isn't a sign of failure. Call your doctor as soon as you have a flare, to ask if your medications need to be changed.

Conclusion

Taking medicines every day can feel tiring, but they are your strongest allies in the fight against lupus nephritis. Each pill is not a punishment but a shield, protecting your kidneys, reducing flares, and preserving your future health. By building simple routines, talking openly with your healthcare team, and seeking support when challenges arise, you can stay on track with your treatment. Remember, it’s normal to face ups and downs — what matters most is consistency, honesty, and partnership with your care team. With the right strategies, medicines can become a source of strength, helping you live fully and confidently with lupus nephritis.

Take home points

- Thoroughly understanding your medications
- Establishing a consistent routine by utilizing reminders like pill organizers, planning refills
- Get regular blood and urine test monitoring
- Know that there are ways to lower your medicine costs
- Building a strong healthcare team that you trust is critical
- Have an open communication with your healthcare team

Remember, the journey of living with lupus and lupus nephritis is like the journey of life, there will be ups and downs. However, downs aren’t a sign of failure. Rather they are a signal to collaborate with your medical team, reassess your current plan, and make necessary adjustments in your medicines. Remember that you got lupus under control the first time, and you will get it under control again!

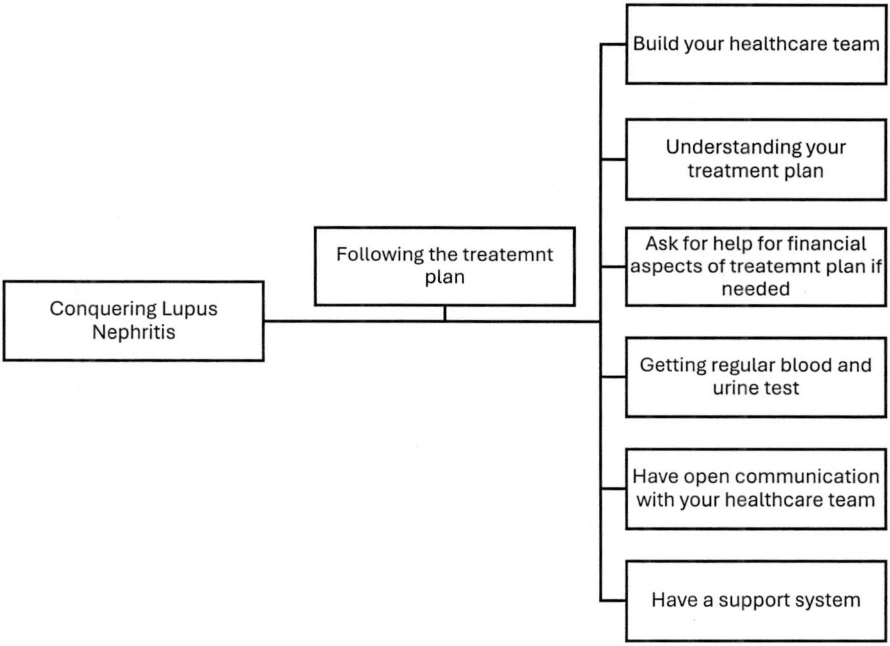

References

1. Ghaussy NO, Sibbitt W, Jr., Bankhurst AD, Qualls CR. The effect of race on disease activity in systemic lupus erythematosus. *J Rheumatol*. May 2004;31(5):915-9.
2. Ward MM. Prevalence of physician-diagnosed systemic lupus erythematosus in the United States: results from the third national health and nutrition examination survey. *J Womens Health (Larchmt)*. Jul-Aug 2004;13(6):713-8. doi:10.1089/jwh.2004.13.713
3. Barr RG, Seliger S, Appel GB, et al. Prognosis in proliferative lupus nephritis: the role of socio-economic status and race/ethnicity. *Nephrol Dial Transplant*. Oct 2003;18(10):2039-46. doi:10.1093/ndt/gfg345
4. Cervera R, Khamashta MA, Font J, et al. Morbidity and mortality in systemic lupus erythematosus during a 10-year period: a comparison of early and late manifestations in a cohort of 1,000 patients. *Medicine (Baltimore)*. Sep 2003;82(5):299-308.

doi:10.1097/01.md.0000091181.93122.55
5. Gladman DD, Urowitz MB, Rahman P, Ibañez D, Tam LS. Accrual of organ damage over time in patients with systemic lupus erythematosus. *J Rheumatol*. Sep 2003;30(9):1955-9.
6. Alarcón GS, McGwin G, Jr., Petri M, Reveille JD, Ramsey-Goldman R, Kimberly RP. Baseline characteristics of a multiethnic lupus cohort: PROFILE. *Lupus*. 2002;11(2):95-101. doi:10.1191/0961203302lu155oa
7. Bastian HM, Roseman JM, McGwin G, Jr., et al. Systemic lupus erythematosus in three ethnic groups. XII. Risk factors for lupus nephritis after diagnosis. *Lupus*. 2002;11(3):152-60. doi:10.1191/0961203302lu158oa
8. Seligman VA, Lum RF, Olson JL, Li H, Criswell LA. Demographic differences in the development of lupus nephritis: a retrospective analysis. *Am J Med*. Jun 15 2002;112(9):726-9. doi:10.1016/s0002-9343(02)01118-x
9. Alarcón GS, McGwin G, Jr., Bastian HM, et al. Systemic lupus erythematosus in three ethnic groups. VII [correction of VIII]. Predictors of early mortality in the LUMINA cohort. LUMINA Study Group. *Arthritis Rheum*. Apr 2001;45(2):191-202. doi:10.1002/1529-0131(200104)45:2<191::aid-anr173>3.0.co;2-2
10. Bruce IN, Gladman DD, Urowitz MB. Factors associated with refractory renal disease in patients with systemic lupus erythematosus: the role of patient nonadherence. *Arthritis Care Res*. Dec 2000;13(6):406-8.
11. Xie SK, Feng SF, Fu H. Long term follow-up of patients with systemic lupus erythematosus. *J Dermatol*. Jun 1998;25(6):367-73. doi:10.1111/j.1346-8138.1998.tb02416.x
12. Pistiner M, Wallace DJ, Nessim S, Metzger AL, Klinenberg JR. Lupus erythematosus in the 1980s: a survey of 570 patients. *Semin Arthritis Rheum*. Aug 1991;21(1):55-64. doi:10.1016/0049-0172(91)90057-7
13. Petri M, Orbai AM, Alarcon GS, et al. Derivation and validation of the Systemic Lupus International Collaborating Clinics classification criteria for systemic lupus erythematosus. *Arthritis Rheum*. Aug 2012;64(8):2677-86. doi:10.1002/art.34473
14. Gladman DD, Ibanez D, Urowitz MB. Systemic lupus erythematosus disease activity index 2000. *J Rheumatol*. Feb 2002;29(2):288-91.
15. Urowitz M, Gladman D, Bruce I. Atherosclerosis and systemic lupus erythematosus. *Curr Rheumatol Rep*. Feb 2000;2(1):19-23.

16. Gladman D, Ginzler E, Goldsmith C, et al. The development and initial validation of the Systemic Lupus International Collaborating Clinics/American College of Rheumatology damage index for systemic lupus erythematosus. *Arthritis Rheum*. Mar 1996;39(3): 363-9. doi:10.1002/art.1780390303
17. Gladman DD. Indicators of disease activity, prognosis, and treatment of systemic lupus erythematosus. *Curr Opin Rheumatol*. Sep 1994;6(5):487-92.
18. Fanouriakis A, Kostopoulou M, Andersen J, et al. EULAR recommendations for the management of systemic lupus erythematosus: 2023 update. *Ann Rheum Dis*. Jan 2 2024;83(1):15-29. doi:10.1136/ard-2023-224762
19. Antonis F, Myrto K, Jeanette A, et al. EULAR recommendations for the management of systemic lupus erythematosus: 2023 update. *Annals of the Rheumatic Diseases*. 2023:ard-2023-224762.
20. Nguyen Y, Blanchet B, Urowitz MB, et al. Association Between Severe Nonadherence to Hydroxychloroquine and Systemic Lupus Erythematosus Flares, Damage, and Mortality in 660 Patients From the SLICC Inception Cohort. *Arthritis Rheumatol*. Dec 2023;75(12): 2195-2206. doi:10.1002/art.42645
21. Almeida-Brasil CC, Hanly JG, Urowitz M, et al. Flares after hydroxychloroquine reduction or discontinuation: results from the Systemic Lupus International Collaborating Clinics (SLICC) inception cohort. *Annals of the Rheumatic Diseases*. 2022;81(3):370. doi:10.1136/annrheumdis-2021-221295
22. Clowse MEB, Eudy AM, Balevic S, et al. Hydroxychloroquine in the pregnancies of women with lupus: a meta-analysis of individual participant data. *Lupus Sci Med*. Mar 2022;9(1)doi:10.1136/lupus-2021-000651
23. Tselios K, Gladman DD, Su J, Urowitz MB. Antimalarials as a risk factor for elevated muscle enzymes in systemic lupus erythematosus. *Lupus*. Apr 2016;25(5):532-5. doi:10.1177/0961203315617845
24. Akhavan PS, Su J, Lou W, Gladman DD, Urowitz MB, Fortin PR. The early protective effect of hydroxychloroquine on the risk of cumulative damage in patients with systemic lupus erythematosus. *J Rheumatol*. Jun 2013;40(6):831-41. doi:10.3899/jrheum.12057210.3899/jrheum.120572. Epub 2013 Apr 15.
25. Steiman AJ, Gladman DD, Ibanez D, Urowitz MB. Outcomes in patients with systemic lupus erythematosus with and without a

prolonged serologically active clinically quiescent period. *Arthritis Care Res (Hoboken)*. Apr 2012;64(4):511-8. doi:10.1002/acr.21568 10.1002/acr.21568.

26. Jung H, Bobba R, Su J, et al. The protective effect of antimalarial drugs on thrombovascular events in systemic lupus erythematosus. *Arthritis Rheum*. Mar 2010;62(3):863-8. doi:10.1002/art.27289 10.1002/art.27289.
27. Tam LS, Gladman DD, Hallett DC, Rahman P, Urowitz MB. Effect of antimalarial agents on the fasting lipid profile in systemic lupus erythematosus. *J Rheumatol*. Sep 2000;27(9):2142-5.
28. Rahman P, Humphrey-Murto S, Gladman DD, Urowitz MB. Efficacy and tolerability of methotrexate in antimalarial resistant lupus arthritis. *J Rheumatol*. Feb 1998;25(2):243-6.
29. Garg S, Rovin B, Astor B, et al. Hydroxychloroquine Users at Lower Risk of Kidney Function Decline in Lupus Nephritis [abstract]. 2024; Accessed Accessed May 18, 2025. https://acrabstracts.org/abstract/hydroxychloroquine-users-at-lower-risk-of-kidney-function-decline-in-lupus-nephritis/.
30. Garg S, Chewning B, Gazeley D, et al. Patient and healthcare team recommended medication adherence strategies for hydroxychloroquine: results of a qualitative study informing intervention development. *Lupus Sci Med*. Aug 2022;9(1)doi:10.1136/lupus-2022-000720
31. Garg S, Patel J, Ferguson S, et al. Clarifying Misbeliefs & Resolving Decisional Conflicts About Hydroxychloroquine (HCQ) Through a Shared Decision-Making Tool (HCQ-SAFE©) [abstract]. Presented at: A*merican College of Rheumatology, Annual Convergence*; 2024; Washington D.C. Accessed Accessed April 8, 2025. https://acrabstracts.org/abstract/clarifying-misbeliefs-resolving-decisional-conflicts-about-hydroxychloroquine-hcq-through-a-shared-decision-making-tool-hcq-safe/.
32. Garg S, Ferguson S, Chewning B, Gomez S, Keevil J, Bartels C. Clarifying misbeliefs about hydroxychloroquine (HCQ): developing the HCQ benefits versus harm decision aid (HCQ-SAFE) per low health literacy standards. *Lupus Sci Med*. Jul 2023;10(2) doi:10.1136/lupus-2023-000935
33. Nasrallah CH, C. Kasturi, S. Machua, W. Yazdany, J. Bartels, CM. Chieseri, K. Blanks, S. Katz, P. Wilson, C. Jorge, A. Radtke, B. Tack, T. Garg, S. *Development of the American College of Rheumatology Implementation Guide for Integrating Patient Reported Systemic Lupus Erythematosus Quality Measures.* presented at: 2025

American College of Rheumatology Convergence; 2025.; Chicago, IL.

34. Sammaritano LR, Askanase A, Bermas BL, et al. 2024 American College of Rheumatology (ACR) Guideline for the Screening, Treatment, and Management of Lupus Nephritis. *Arthritis Rheumatol.* May 7 2025;doi:10.1002/art.43212
35. Bartels CM, Jorge A, Feldman CH, et al. Development of American College of Rheumatology Quality Measures for Systemic Lupus Erythematosus: A Modified Delphi Process With Rheumatology Informatics System for Effectiveness (RISE) Registry Data Review. *Arthritis Care & Research*. 2023/05/11 2023;n/a(n/a) doi:https://doi.org/10.1002/acr.25143
36. Petri M. Drug monitoring in systemic lupus erythematosus. *Curr Opin Pharmacol*. Jun 2022;64:102225. doi:10.1016/j.coph.2022.102225
37. Garg S, Chewning B, Hutson P, Astor BC, Bartels CM. Reference Range of Hydroxychloroquine Blood Levels That Can Reduce Odds of Active Lupus and Prevent Flares. *Arthritis Care Res (Hoboken)*. Feb 2024;76(2):241-250. doi:10.1002/acr.25228
38. Garg S, Astor BC, Saric C, et al. Therapeutic Hydroxychloroquine Blood Levels Are Associated With Fewer Hospitalizations and Possible Reduction of Health Disparities in Lupus. *Arthritis Care Res (Hoboken)*. Dec 2024;76(12):1606-1616. doi:10.1002/acr.25422
39. Garg S, Chewning B, Astor B, Bartels C. Therapeutic Thresholds of Hydroxychloroquine Blood Levels: Physiologic and Social Determinants of Low Hydroxychloroquine Blood Levels [abstract]. . *2022*; Accessed Accessed September 14, 2022. https://acrabstracts.org/abstract/therapeutic-thresholds-of-hydroxychloroquine-blood-levels-physiologic-and-social-determinants-of-low-hydroxychloroquine-blood-levels/.
40. Garg S, Unnithan R, Hansen KE, Costedoat-Chalumeau N, Bartels CM. Clinical Significance of Monitoring Hydroxychloroquine Levels in Patients With Systemic Lupus Erythematosus: A Systematic Review and Meta-Analysis. *Arthritis Care Res (Hoboken)*. May 2021;73(5):707-716. doi:10.1002/acr.24155
41. Lenfant T, Costedoat-Chalumeau N. Hydroxychloroquine dose: balancing toxicity and SLE flare risk. *Nat Rev Rheumatol*. Jan 2023;19(1):6-7. doi:10.1038/s41584-022-00868-3
42. Lenfant T, Salah S, Leroux G, et al. Risk factors for hydroxychloroquine retinopathy in systemic lupus erythematosus: a case-control study

with hydroxychloroquine blood-level analysis. *Rheumatology (Oxford, England)*. 2020/12// 2020;59(12):3807-3816. doi:10.1093/rheumatology/keaa157

43. Costedoat-Chalumeau N, Isenberg D, Petri M. Comment on the 2019 update of the EULAR recommendations for the management of systemic lupus erythematosus by Fanouriakis et al. *Ann Rheum Dis*. 2020:e90. vol. 8.
44. Costedoat-Chalumeau N, Tamirou F, Le Guern V, Blanchet B, Deligny C, Piette JC. [Blood concentration of hydroxychloroquine in systemic lupus erythematosus care: Usefulness and limits]. *Rev Med Interne*. Feb 2017;38(2):77-80. Dosage sanguin de l'hydroxychloroquine dans la prise en charge du lupus systemique : interets et limites. doi:10.1016/j.revmed.2016.07.001 10.1016/j.revmed.2016.07.001. Epub 2016 Oct 13.
45. Chasset F, Bouaziz JD, Costedoat-Chalumeau N, Francès C, Arnaud L. Efficacy and comparison of antimalarials in cutaneous lupus erythematosus subtypes: a systematic review and meta-analysis. *Br J Dermatol*. Jul 2017;177(1):188-196. doi:10.1111/bjd.15312
46. Costedoat-Chalumeau N, Houssiau F, Izmirly P, et al. A Prospective International Study on Adherence to Treatment in 305 Patients With Flaring SLE: Assessment by Drug Levels and Self-Administered Questionnaires. *Clin Pharmacol Ther*. Jun 2017;103(6):1074-1082. doi:10.1002/cpt.885 10.1002/cpt.885. Epub 2017 Nov 9.
47. Qu Y, Noe G, Breaud AR, et al. Development and validation of a clinical HPLC method for the quantification of hydroxychloroquine and its metabolites in whole blood. *Future Sci OA*. Nov 2015;1(3):Fso26. doi:10.4155/fso.15.24
48. Costedoat-Chalumeau N, V LEG, Piette JC. Routine Hydroxychloroquine Blood Concentration Measurement in Systemic Lupus Erythematosus Reaches Adulthood. *J Rheumatol*. Nov 2015;42(11):1997-9. doi:10.3899/jrheum.151094
49. Francès C, Cosnes A, Duhaut P, et al. Low blood concentration of hydroxychloroquine in patients with refractory cutaneous lupus erythematosus: a French multicenter prospective study. *Arch Dermatol*. Apr 2012;148(4):479-84. doi:10.1001/archdermatol.2011.2558
50. Izmirly PM, Costedoat-Chalumeau N, Pisoni CN, et al. Maternal use of hydroxychloroquine is associated with a reduced risk of recurrent anti-SSA/Ro-antibody-associated cardiac manifestations of neonatal lupus. *Circulation*. Jul 3 2012;126(1):76-82. doi:10.1161/circulationaha.111.089268

51. Costedoat-Chalumeau N, Amoura Z, Hulot J-S, et al. Very low blood hydroxychloroquine concentration as an objective marker of poor adherence to treatment of systemic lupus erythematosus. *Annals of the Rheumatic Diseases*. Jun 2007;66(6):821-824. doi:10.1136/ard.2006.067835
52. Costedoat-Chalumeau N, Amoura Z, Hulot JS, et al. Low blood concentration of hydroxychloroquine is a marker for and predictor of disease exacerbations in patients with systemic lupus erythematosus. *Arthritis Rheum*. Oct 2006;54(10):3284-90. doi:10.1002/art.22156
53. Petri M, Konig MF, Li J, Goldman DW. Association of Higher Hydroxychloroquine Blood Levels With Reduced Thrombosis Risk in Systemic Lupus Erythematosus. *Arthritis Rheumatol*. Jun 2021;73(6):997-1004. doi:10.1002/art.41621
54. Petri M, Elkhalifa M, Li J, Magder LS, Goldman DW. Hydroxychloroquine Blood Levels Predict Hydroxychloroquine Retinopathy. *Arthritis Rheumatol*. Mar 2020;72(3):448-453. doi:10.1002/art.41121
55. Durcan L, Winegar DA, Connelly MA, Otvos JD, Magder LS, Petri M. Longitudinal Evaluation of Lipoprotein Variables in Systemic Lupus Erythematosus Reveals Adverse Changes with Disease Activity and Prednisone and More Favorable Profiles with Hydroxychloroquine Therapy. *J Rheumatol*. Apr 2016;43(4):745-50. doi:10.3899/jrheum.150437
56. Garg S, Chewning B, Gazeley D, et al. Patient and healthcare team recommended medication adherence strategies for hydroxychloroquine: results of a qualitative study informing intervention development. *Lupus Science & Medicine*. 2022;9(1):e000720. doi:10.1136/lupus-2022-000720
57. Garg S, Singh T, Panzer SE, Astor BC, Bartels CM. Multidisciplinary Lupus Nephritis Clinic Reduces Time to Renal Biopsy and Improves Care Quality. *ACR Open Rheumatol*. Jul 2022;4(7):581-586. doi:10.1002/acr2.11435

CHAPTER 7

EATING FOR KIDNEY HEALTH

NOURISHING CHOICES THAT SUPPORT YOUR BODY DAILY

MANSI JAIN
DEPARTMENT OF INTERNAL MEDICINE,
ST. VINCENT MEDICAL CENTER TOLEDO, OHIO

Abstract

Nutrition plays a vital role in supporting people with lupus nephritis, working hand in hand with medications to protect the kidneys and improve overall well-being. This chapter explores how thoughtful food choices can reduce inflammation, manage blood pressure, preserve bone and heart health, and prevent complications such as anemia. It provides practical guidance on macronutrients — balancing proteins, fats, and carbohydrates — and explains how to choose foods that are easier on the kidneys. Key micronutrients such as sodium, potassium, phosphorus, calcium, vitamin D, iron, and folic acid are highlighted with tips for managing their intake safely. Emerging research on probiotics and plant-based antioxidants is also discussed as promising tools for kidney health. By learning how to adapt everyday meals, patients can use nutrition as a powerful partner in their lupus nephritis care plan, supporting both energy and long-term kidney function.

Keywords: Lupus Nephritis, Nutrition, Kidney Health, Inflammation, Micronutrients.

Let's start this chapter with the hypothetical story of Sofia. Sofia stood in the grocery aisle, holding a package of bacon in one hand and a bag of fresh vegetables in the other. Before her diagnosis of lupus nephritis, the choice would have been easy — bacon was her comfort food, quick and tasty. But now, she thought about the swelling in her legs, the long hospital stays, and the doctor's words about how her kidneys needed protection.

She paused, remembering how tired she had felt when her blood pressure soared and how helpless it seemed when her labs showed worsening kidney function. Back then, food was just food. Now, every bite felt like a decision for her future.

Slowly, she put the bacon back and reached for the vegetables. She imagined cooking a simple stir-fry with olive oil, garlic, and fresh greens. It wasn't about giving up everything she enjoyed — it was about learning new ways to nourish her body.

As she pushed her cart down the aisle, Sofia realized nutrition wasn't a restriction but an opportunity. Each meal she prepared was a chance to care for her kidneys, reduce inflammation, and live with more energy. For Sofia, food had become more than fuel; it was a powerful partner in her healing journey.

Like Sofia, many people with lupus nephritis discover that small, everyday food choices can make a big difference in protecting their kidneys and improving their overall health.

Managing lupus nephritis can feel overwhelming, but your plate holds more power than you might think. While medications are essential in controlling disease activity, nutrition can be a key partner in your treatment plan. A well-balanced diet helps reduce inflammation, control blood pressure, prevent complications like bone loss and anemia, and support energy levels.

This chapter will offer practical and easy-to-understand dietary recommendations tailored for people living with lupus nephritis. From macronutrients like proteins, fats, and carbohydrates to essential vitamins and minerals, each section provides information to help you make choices that align with your medical needs. Whether you are just diagnosed or managing lupus nephritis long-term, a thoughtful and balanced diet will improve your health and quality of life.

Plant-Based vs Animal-Based Diet:

Recent studies suggest that increasing your intake of whole plant-based foods, such as fruits, vegetables, beans, nuts, and whole grains, can help protect your kidneys. This type of eating pattern, known as a whole food plant-based diet, may slow kidney damage, reduce inflammation, and even delay the need for dialysis [1]. Plant based foods are generally gentler on the kidneys compared to animal proteins like red meat, which can produce more acid and place additional stress on the body and kidneys. However, it is important to ensure you are still meeting your protein and nutrient needs, so working with a licensed kidney dietitian is a wise choice. Your kidney doctor can refer you to a licensed kidney dietitian.

One well known variation of a plant-based diet is the Mediterranean diet, which has also shown positive impact on health in people with lupus nephritis. This diet emphasizes olive oil, vegetables, fruits, legumes, whole grains, and fish, and has been shown to reduce inflammation and lower the risk of cardiovascular disease, an important benefit as people with lupus are at high risk for heart problems [2].

Macronutrients

Macronutrients such as proteins, fats, and carbohydrates are the foundation of your daily diet. But in lupus nephritis, the type and amount of each macronutrient matters. This section will walk you through how to choose these nutrients wisely to support kidney health, reduce inflammation, and maintain strength and energy.

1. Proteins:

Proteins are like the bricks that help build and repair your body, from your muscles to your bones. They also give you energy and help you stay strong.

But here is the catch: when your body breaks down extra or old proteins, it creates waste products like urea and other uremic toxins. These normally get filtered out by your kidneys and flushed away in your urine. If your kidneys aren't working well, this “waste pile” starts building up. And that can lead to problems like weakness, nausea, confusion, or even inflammation of the heart and lungs.

So, does this mean you should stop eating protein? Not at all! The key is balance: just enough protein to keep you strong, but not so much that your kidneys give up.

According to the guidelines, your protein needs depend on how well your kidneys are working [3,4].

Protein Intake Recommendations - It depends on degree of kidney dysfunction

Kidney Function	Recommended Protein intake
CKD Grade 1 to Grade 2	0.8 to 1.0 g/kg/day
CKD Grade 3 to Grade 5	0.6 to 0.8 g/kg/day
ESRD on dialysis	1.0 to 1.2 g/kg/day (due to protein loss during dialysis)

CKD: Chronic Kidney Disease; ESRD: End Stage Renal Disease

High protein diets (more than 1.3 g/kg/day) are not recommended due to the risk of worsening kidney function [3]. Diets lower than 0.6 g/kg/day are not routinely recommended due to risk of malnutrition [3].

What Type of Proteins?

So, which proteins get a thumbs up? Plant based ones win the gold star.

Studies show that they may help slow kidney disease and even lower your chances of dying from kidney related problems [5,6]. Plant based diets produce less waste, contain less phosphorus (which can hurt your bones and heart), and are packed with good things like antioxidants, fiber, and polyphenols. All that helps reduce inflammation, which is especially important in lupus.

Protein Sources

Category	Examples	Clinical Guidance
Plant Based Proteins	Lentils, chickpeas, black beans, kidney beans	Preferred sources; lower phosphorus bioavailability and acid load
	Tofu, tempeh, edamame, soy milk	High quality plant proteins with full amino acid profiles
	Quinoa, oats, brown rice, barley	Combine with legumes for complete proteins

	Almonds, walnuts, flaxseeds, chia seeds	High in healthy fats; limit portion size due to potassium and phosphorus content
Animal Based Proteins	Egg whites, whole eggs (moderation)	Egg whites preferred for low phosphorus; whole eggs in moderation
	Salmon, tuna, sardines, tilapia, shrimp	Rich in omega 3; anti-inflammatory benefits; lower saturated fat
	Skinless chicken breast, turkey	Lean protein; limit portions to reduce acid and nitrogen burden
	Low fat dairy (Greek yogurt, milk, cottage cheese)	Acceptable in moderate amounts; watch phosphorus and potassium
To Limit or Avoid	Red meats (beef, lamb, pork)	High acid load and phosphorus; associated with faster CKD progression
	Processed meats (sausage, bacon, salami, deli meats)	High sodium, nitrates, and phosphorus additives; linked to inflammation
	High sodium meats (smoked fish, canned meats, meat jerky)	Contribute to fluid retention and hypertension; increase cardiovascular risk
	Organ meats (liver, kidney, sweetbreads)	High in purines and phosphorus; not recommended in kidney disease

Tips for Protein Intake:

- **Know your number:** Ask your doctor or dietitian how much protein you need each day (usually 0.6 to 0.8 g/kg for non-dialysis patients).
- **Go plant based when possible:** Beans, lentils, tofu, and nuts are great choices.
- **Pick lean animal proteins:** If you eat meat, go for egg whites, fish, or skinless chicken.
- **Avoid red and processed meats:** Limit beef, pork, bacon, sausages, and deli meats, they stress your kidneys and raise inflammation.
- **Pair your proteins:** Foods like rice and beans or hummus and whole grain bread make complete proteins together.
- **Choose healthy cooking methods:** Bake, grill, steam, or stew. Skip the deep fryer.

2. Fats:

Despite their bad reputation, not all fats are villains. In fact, some are essential heroes, especially when it comes to protecting your heart and kidneys [7]. For people with lupus nephritis, where the risk of heart disease is higher, choosing the right kind of fat is more important than ever.

So, let's decode the fat family. Who's got your back and who's quietly clogging your arteries?

Natural Fats

Natural fats come from foods we know and recognize, but not all of them play nice inside the body.

- **Saturated fats** – These are the old school fats that stay solid at room temperature. Think butter, ghee, the fat on red meat. Chemically, they are "full," saturated with hydrogen, and they can stiffen your arteries over time. Best to keep these on the occasional guest list, not in your daily rotation.

Common sources:

1. Butter
2. Lard
3. Red meat fat
4. Cheese
5. Palm and coconut oil

- **Unsaturated fats** – These are the flexible, heart friendly fats that stay liquid at room temperature. Their structure has gaps called double bonds that make them better for your body.

Two types:

1. **Monounsaturated fats (MUFA)** – Found in olive oil, avocados, almonds, and peanuts
2. **Polyunsaturated fats (PUFA)** – Found in sunflower oil, flaxseed, walnuts, and fatty fishlike salmon

These are beneficial and try to include them often.

Artificial Fats

- **Trans fats** are man-made fats. They're made by forcing hydrogen into vegetable oil to make it solid. Great for shelf life, terrible for your heart.

Sources:

1. Packaged baked goods (cookies, crackers, cakes)
2. Fried fast food
3. Stick margarine
4. Vanaspati ghee

Even in small amounts, trans fats are linked to a higher risk of heart disease [8]. Always check the label even if it says, "0 g trans-fat". Scan for the words "partially hydrogenated oils."

So, How Much Fat Is Just Right?

You don't have to fear fat, but you do need to be smart about it. It is recommended [9]:

1. Total fat: 25 to 35% of your daily calories
2. Saturated fat: Less than 7%
3. Trans fat: Less than 1%
4. Monounsaturated fat (MUFA): Up to 20%
5. Polyunsaturated fat (PUFA): Up to 10%

Tips for Fat Intake:

Incorporating healthier fats into daily meals can be achieved through simple and practical substitutions:

- Replace butter or ghee with oils such as olive, sunflower, or flaxseed for cooking and dressings.
- Favor grilling, roasting, or baking over deep frying to reduce saturated fat intake.
- Add ground flaxseeds to oatmeal, yogurt, or smoothies for a source of beneficial omega 3 fatty acids.
- Use avocado or hummus in place of mayonnaise as a nutrient dense spread.
- Consider tahini or blended cashew paste as alternatives for creating creamy sauces or dips.
- **Choose oils over butter** – Cook with olive, sunflower, or flaxseed oil instead of ghee or butter.
- **Snack smart** – Reach for a handful of almonds, a spoonful of peanut butter, or slices of avocado.
- **Limit red meat and full fat dairy** – Opt for skinless chicken, beans, or low-fat yogurt.
- **Avoid packaged fried foods** – Say no to doughnuts, frozen fries, or anything that lists "hydrogenated oil."
- **Read food labels carefully** – Don't let "0 g trans-fat" fool you. Double check the ingredients.

3. Carbohydrates:

Carbohydrates are the body's primary source of energy, breaking down into glucose to fuel your cells. But like any fuel, the type and quantity matter. Too much of the wrong kind can lead to trouble. Obesity, for instance, has been linked to increased inflammation in people with lupus [10]. Moreover, many patients with lupus take steroids either during flare ups or long term, their risk of developing diabetes is already higher.

So, what kinds of carbohydrates should you include, and which ones should you limit or avoid?

1. Low Glycemic Index (GI) Carbohydrates:

The glycemic index (GI) measures how quickly a food raises your blood sugar after you eat it. Low GI foods cause a slower, steadier rise in blood sugar. This helps prevent spikes of sugar that can increase inflammation and worsen lupus symptoms. There has been some evidence that low GI foods may improve quality of life in people with lupus [11].

Sources:

- Legumes: Lentils, chickpeas, black beans
- Whole grains: Barley, quinoa, steel cut oats
- Fruits: Apples, pears, berries
- Vegetables: Sweet potato, carrots
- Dairy: Milk, yogurt (unsweetened)

2. High Glycemic Index (GI) Carbohydrates:

High GI foods are absorbed quickly and cause rapid spikes in blood sugar. These spikes can trigger inflammation and increase the risk of diabetes. They also lead to a quick crash in energy, often making you feel hungry again soon after eating.

Sources to limit or avoid:

- White bread, white rice
- Instant oats
- Sugar sweetened cereals
- Potatoes (especially mashed or baked without skin)
- Pastries, cakes, soda, candy

3. Complex Carbohydrates

These carbs are made of long chains of sugar molecules and are usually digested more slowly. Many complex carbs also have a low or moderate glycemic index, but not always.

Sources:

- Whole grains: Brown rice, whole wheat bread, bulgur
- Vegetables: Broccoli, spinach, carrots
- Legumes: Beans, lentils, peas
- Tubers: Sweet potatoes, yams

Key Point: Complex ≠ always low GI. For example, instant oatmeal is technically a complex carb but has a high GI. Choose complex carbs that are also low GI when possible.

Smart Swaps:

Avoid	Replace With
White Rice	Brown rice or Quinoa
White Bread	100% whole wheat or sprouted bread
Sugary cereal	Oatmeal with Cinnamon and Berries
Potato Chips	Air popped popcorn or roasted chickpeas
Soda	Water with lemon, herbal tea

How Much Carbohydrate Should You Eat?

For patients with kidney disease, especially those on a protein restricted diet, carbohydrates should provide approximately 45% to 65% of total energy intake [12].

Take home message:

Total Calorie Intake – Dietary energy provision for both dialysis and non-dialysis CKD patients should be 30 to 35 kcal/kg (ideal body weight) per day [13].

Nutrient	Recommended Intake	Recommended Source
Carbohydrates	45-60% of total energy	Low Gl carbohydrates preferred over High GI
Proteins	0.6-0.8 g/kg/day (adjusted per CKD Stage)	Whole plant-based proteins preferred over animal proteins
Fats	Approximately 25-30% of total energy	Unsaturated fats preferred over saturated and trans fats

Micronutrients:

While macronutrients form the bulk of your diet, micronutrients like sodium, potassium, phosphorus, calcium, and iron play equally vital roles. When kidney function is impaired, even small amounts of these minerals can have a big impact. The next section explains which ones to watch closely and how to manage them through smart food choices.

1. Sodium:

Sodium (commonly known as salt) is essential for the body, but when you have lupus nephritis or chronic kidney disease, too much sodium can cause problems. If your kidneys are not working well, they may not be able to remove excess sodium, leading to fluid buildup, swelling, and high blood pressure, all of which place extra stress on your kidneys and heart.

The current guideline recommends limiting sodium intake to less than 2 grams per day, which is about 5 grams of salt, or roughly one teaspoon per day from all sources, not just the salt you add at the table [3].

You might be surprised to learn that most sodium in your diet comes from packaged foods, processed snacks, and restaurant meals, not just the saltshaker.

High Sodium Foods	**Healthier Choices**
Canned Soup/Veggies	Low sodium versions or rinse before eating
Packaged snacks and chips	Air popped popcorn, unsalted nuts
Pickles, olives and condiments	Fresh veggies, herbs and vinegar
Instant noodles or ramen	Homemade soups using herbs and lemon
Sauces (soy, BBQ etc.)	Make your own with minimal salt
Bread and baked goods	Check labels, many processed foods add salt
Restaurant meals	Ask for no-salt added options

2. Potassium:

Healthy kidneys help regulate potassium levels by removing the excess through urine. In kidney disease, the kidneys may not clear potassium efficiently, leading to elevated levels. High potassium can cause muscle weakness, irregular heart rhythms, or even cardiac arrest if severe.

That's why your kidney doctor regularly checks your potassium and other electrolyte levels. If your potassium is high, you may be advised to follow a low-potassium diet. It's helpful to know which foods are high in potassium and which ones are safer options.

Potassium Content in Common Foods

Food Category	High Potassium Foods	Low Potassium Foods
Fruits	Bananas, oranges, avocados, cantaloupe, kiwis, dried fruits	Apples, grapes, berries, pineapple
Vegetables	Potatoes, sweet potatoes, tomatoes, spinach, beet greens, pumpkin	Green beans, cabbage, cauliflower, lettuce, eggplant
Dairy	Milk, yogurt, ice cream	Rice Milk (unenriched), almond milk (low potassium type)
Proteins	Beans, lentils, nuts, seeds	Small amount of chicken, egg whites, tofu (in moderation)
Starches/grains	Bran cereals, whole grains (in excess)	White rice, pasta, white bread, low potassium cereals
Snacks/Other	Chocolate, molasses, coconut water	Popcorn (unsalted), plain crackers, short bread cookies

3. Phosphorus:

Phosphorus plays an important role in keeping our bones and teeth strong. Normally, healthy kidneys remove excess phosphorus through urine. But in kidney disease, the kidneys may not filter it effectively, leading to **phosphorus buildup in the blood**.

Why does that matter? When phosphorus levels are too high, it pulls calcium out of the bones to form calcium-phosphate crystals, making bones weak and prone to fractures. Moreover, these crystals can deposit in blood vessels, hardening them and increasing the risk of heart disease.

That's why your kidney doctor regularly monitors your phosphorus levels. If your phosphorus is high, you may be advised to follow a low-phosphorus diet.

Common Food Sources of Phosphorus

Category	High-Phosphorus Foods to Limit	Lower-Phosphorus Alternatives
Dairy	Cheese, milk, ice cream	Small amounts of cream cheese, rice milk, almond milk
Meats	Organ meats (liver), processed meats	Fresh poultry, egg whites
Grains	Whole grain bread, bran cereal	White rice, white bread, low-phosphorus cereal (cornflakes)
Packaged Foods	Colas, bottled iced teas, fast foods, processed cheese	Water, lemon water, homemade snacks
Additives	Anything with "phos-" ingredients on label	Choose fresh, homemade, or label-free foods

One of the biggest sources of phosphorus to be aware of is phosphorus from preservatives or additives. This type of phosphorus is in inorganic form, which is absorbed almost 90–100% by the body [14]. In contrast, only 40–60% of natural phosphorus (found in beans, nuts, or whole grains) is absorbed [14].

Added phosphorus is not always easy to spot. It hides under ingredient names like:

- Sodium phosphate
- Calcium phosphate
- Phosphoric acid
- Dicalcium phosphate

Tips to Low Phosphorus:

- Read ingredient labels and avoid items with **"phos-"** in the name (e.g., phosphoric acid).
- **Limit dairy** and choose low-phosphorus plant-based options like almond or rice milk.
- **Avoid cola and dark sodas**, which often contain added phosphates.
- **Choose fresh foods over processed ones**, since processed and packaged foods tend to have phosphate additives.
- If your levels remain high, your doctor may prescribe medications called **phosphate binders** to reduce phosphorus absorption from food.

4. Calcium and Vitamin D:

Calcium and vitamin D are essential nutrients that work together to keep our bones strong and healthy. In healthy individuals, the kidneys help activate vitamin D, which in turn increases calcium absorption from the gut and reduces calcium loss through the urine. This allows calcium to deposit into the bones, strengthening them and reducing the risk of fractures.

However, chronic kidney disease (CKD), the kidneys lose their ability to activate vitamin D effectively. This leads to lower calcium absorption, weaker bones, and a higher risk of fractures. The problem is made worse in lupus patients who are often on long-term steroids which further weaken bones and who may avoid sunlight due to photosensitivity, resulting in lower natural vitamin D production.

Because of these risks, kidney doctors regularly check your vitamin D and calcium levels. If needed, they may recommend dietary adjustments or supplements to help maintain bone health and prevent complications.

Common Food sources of Calcium and Vitamin D

Nutrient	**Better Food Sources**	**Tips**
Calcium	Fortified almond milk, rice milk, tofu, leafy greens (collard greens, kale), canned salmon with bones	Avoid excess dairy if phosphorus is high
Vitamin D	Fortified cereals and plant milks, fatty fish (salmon, sardines), eggs	Safe sunlight exposure can help your body produce vitamin D

5. Iron and Folic Acid:

Anemia, or low red blood cell count, is common in people with lupus nephritis and chronic kidney disease. It can make you feel tired, weak, short of breath, or dizzy. Two key nutrients that help prevent or treat anemia are iron and folic acid.

Normally, the kidneys produce a hormone called erythropoietin (EPO), which signals the body to make red blood cells. But in kidney disease, EPO production drops, resulting in fewer red blood cells, a condition called anemia.

Iron is needed to make hemoglobin, the oxygen-carrying part of red blood cells. In lupus, chronic inflammation can interfere with iron's ability to form hemoglobin, leading to anemia.

Folic acid also supports red blood cell production. Many lupus patients take immunosuppressive medications like methotrexate, which can lower folic acid levels and contribute to anemia.

Common Food Sources of Iron and Folic acid:

Nutrient	Better Food Sources	Tips
Iron	Lean meats, eggs, tofu, lentils, spinach, fortified cereals	Pair with vitamin C rich foods (like citrus or bell peppers) to improve absorption
Folic Acid	Leafy greens, lentils, beans, oranges, fortified cereals	Cooking may reduce folate. Steam or lightly cook vegetables when possible

Tips to Boost Iron:

- Avoid tea or coffee with meals, they can block iron absorption.
- Cook in cast iron pans, it can increase the iron content of food.

Promising Research Areas in Nutrition and Lupus Nephritis

Recent research has started exploring some exciting new areas in nutrition for lupus nephritis, especially around gut health and antioxidant-rich foods. One promising area is probiotics, live bacteria that help maintain a healthy gut microbiome. Some early studies show that probiotics may lower uremic toxins and inflammation in chronic kidney disease [15].

Another group of beneficial compounds is flavonoids, natural plant compounds found in colorful fruits, vegetables, teas, and dark chocolate. These compounds act as antioxidants and may help reduce inflammation, improve blood vessel function, and support immune health in kidney disease [16]. Flavonoids like curcumin (found in turmeric) have shown potential to reduce kidney inflammation in lupus models, although more research is still needed [17].

Conclusion

A thoughtful, kidney-friendly diet can make a real difference in managing lupus nephritis. By focusing on the right balance of macronutrients such as plant-based proteins, complex carbohydrates with low glycemic index, and healthy fats while paying close attention to essential micronutrients like calcium, vitamin D, iron, folic acid, and limiting excessive ones like phosphorus, sodium, and potassium, you can help protect your kidneys and overall health. Emerging research into probiotics and flavonoids offers new hope for enhancing gut health and reducing inflammation. Always work with your healthcare team and dietitian to customize a diet that fits your unique medical needs and lifestyle. Small, consistent dietary choices can empower you to live well with lupus nephritis.

Take home points

- Food can support your kidneys alongside medicines.
- Choose more plant-based proteins and fewer red or processed meats.
- Use healthy fats like olive oil, nuts, and fish instead of butter or fried foods.
- Pick whole grains, fruits, and vegetables with a low glycemic index.
- Limit salt, potassium, and phosphorus to protect your kidneys and heart.

References

(1) Adair KE, Bowden RG. The plant-based diet and chronic kidney disease: A review. J Ren Nutr. 2020;30(6):500-505. Doi: 10.1053/j.jrn.2020.02.007

(2) Pocovi-Gerardino G, Argilés À, Carrasco S, et al. Mediterranean diet adherence in systemic lupus erythematosus patients and its association with disease activity, cardiovascular risk, and quality of life. Nutrients. 2021;13(2):597. doi:10.3390/nu13020597

(3) Kidney Disease: Improving Global Outcomes (KDIGO) CKD Work Group. KDIGO 2024 Clinical Practice Guideline for the Evaluation and Management of Chronic Kidney Disease. *Kidney Int.* 2024;105(4S): S117-S314. Doi: 10.1016/j.kint.2023.10.018

(4) Ikizler TA, Burrowes JD, Byham Gray LD, et al. KDOQI clinical practice guideline for nutrition in CKD: 2020 update. Am J Kidney Dis. 2020;76(3) (suppl 1): S1 to S107.
Doi: 10.1053/j.ajkd.2020.05.006

(5) Bernier Jean A, Prince RL, Lewis JR, et al. Dietary plant and animal protein intake and decline in estimated glomerular filtration rate among elderly women: a 10-year longitudinal cohort study. Nephrol Dial Transplant. 2021;36(9):1640 to 1647. doi:10.1093/ndt/gfaa081

(6) Chen X, Wei G, Jalili T, et al. The Associations of Plant Protein Intake with All-Cause Mortality in CKD. Am J Kidney Dis. 2016;67(3):423 to 430. Doi: 10.1053/j.ajkd.2015.10.018

(7) Lauretani F, Semba RD, Bandinelli S, et al. Plasma polyunsaturated fatty acids and the decline of renal function. Clin Chem. 2008;54(3):475 to 481. doi:10.1373/clinchem.2007.095521

(8) Iqbal MP. Trans fatty acids: A risk factor for cardiovascular disease. Pak J Med Sci. 2014;30(1):194 to 197. doi:10.12669/pjms.301.4525

(9) Kochan Z, Szupryczynska N, Malgorzewicz S, Karbowska J. Dietary Lipids and Dyslipidemia in Chronic Kidney Disease. Nutrients. 2021;13(9):3138. doi:10.3390/nu13093138

(10) Islam MA, Khandker SS, Kotyla PJ, Hassan R. Immunomodulatory effects of diet and nutrients in Systemic Lupus erythematosus (SLE): a systematic review. *Frontiers in Immunology*. 2020;11. doi:10.3389/fimmu.2020.01477

(11) Imoto AM, Gottems LB, Salomon AL, et al. The impact of a low-calorie, low-glycemic diet on systemic lupus erythematosus: a systematic review. *Advances in Rheumatology*. 2021;61(1). doi:10.1186/s42358-021-00224-1

(12) Academy of Nutrition and Dietetics. *Clinical Guide to Nutrition Care in Kidney Disease.* 3rd ed. Chicago, IL: Academy of Nutrition and Dietetics; 2020.

(13) Zha Y, Qian Q. Protein Nutrition and Malnutrition in CKD and ESRD. *Nutrients*. 2017;9(3):208. Published 2017 Feb 27. doi:10.3390/nu9030208

(14) Kalantar-Zadeh K, Gutekunst L, Mehrotra R, et al. Understanding sources of dietary phosphorus in the treatment of patients with chronic kidney disease. *Clin J Am Soc Nephrol.* 2010;5(3):519-530. doi:10.2215/CJN.06080809

(15) Liu W, Li X, Li Y, et al. Effect of probiotic treatment on uremic toxins and inflammation in chronic kidney disease: A systematic review and meta-analysis. Ren Fail. 2020;42(1):1232-1245. doi:10.1080/0886022X.2020.1832806

(16) Cao YL, Lin JH, Hammes HP, Zhang C. Flavonoids in Treatment of Chronic Kidney Disease. *Molecules*. 2022;27(7):2365. Published 2022 Apr 6. doi:10.3390/molecules27072365

(17) Yang F, Lim SC, Li XX, et al. Curcumin as a Therapeutic Candidate for Renal Diseases. Front Pharmacol. 2022; 13:844783. doi:10.3389/fphar.2022.844783

CHAPTER 8

PREGNANCY AND LUPUS NEPHRITIS

WHAT TO KNOW WHEN PLANNING A FAMILY WITH LUPUS

ZOHREH GHOLIZADEH GHOZLOUJEH
AND SAYNA NOROUZI
LOMA LINDA UNIVERSITY

Fertility in Lupus Nephritis: Preserving Your Chances of Pregnancy

If you have lupus nephritis (LN), you may wonder how your condition or its treatments might affect your ability to have children. The good news is that many people with LN can have healthy pregnancies, but planning is key.

This chapter will help you understand how lupus and its treatments can affect fertility, details about birth control and how to have a safe and healthy pregnancy.

How Lupus Nephritis and Its Treatment Affect Fertility

Lupus nephritis is a form of lupus that affects the kidneys. While lupus nephritis itself doesn't always cause fertility problems, some treatments used to manage lupus nephritis can affect fertility. That's why it's important to talk with your doctor before starting any new medication if you plan for pregnancy in future.

Here's how your fertility may be affected:

- **Active disease flares**: Flares of lupus or lupus nephritis can stress the body, and this may impact hormone levels or delay your menstrual cycle. Long-term inflammation may also affect your reproductive health.
- **Medications**: Some medicines used to treat LN, especially cyclophosphamide (Cytoxan), can harm your ovaries and lower your egg count. This is called *ovarian toxicity* and can lead to early menopause or infertility. Other medications like prednisone, used to decrease inflammation, don't usually cause infertility, but high doses over time may affect your menstrual cycle.
- **Age and disease duration**: The longer you've had lupus nephritis and the older you are when starting treatment, the higher the risk of reduced fertility in future

When to Consider Fertility Preservation

If you're thinking about pregnancy in the future, talk to your doctor before starting medications like cyclophosphamide. Fertility preservation is most effective when planned.

You may want to consider fertility preservation if:

- You are about to start a medication known to affect fertility.
- You are in remission and want to delay pregnancy for personal or medical reasons.
- You're unsure about the timing of future pregnancies but want to keep your options open.

Fertility Preservation Options

There are safe and effective ways to preserve fertility:

1. Egg Freezing (Oocyte Cryopreservation)

- Involves collecting eggs after hormone treatment and freezing them for future use.
- Best done before starting gonadotoxic medications like cyclophosphamide.
- Safe in lupus patients if the disease is stable. Your doctor may adjust the hormone stimulation to avoid flares.

2. Embryo Freezing

- Similar to egg freezing, but the egg is fertilized with sperm before being frozen.
- Requires a sperm donor or partner.
- This may be a good option for couples planning future pregnancies.

3. Ovarian Suppression with Hormonal Injections

- Medications like GnRH agonists (e.g., leuprolide) may help protect the ovaries during treatment.
- These are given as injections before and during cyclophosphamide treatment.
- While not as reliable as egg freezing, this is a common method for reducing risk of damage.

4. Ovarian Tissue Freezing

- A newer and more complex option that involves removing and freezing ovarian tissue.
- Less common but may be considered in younger patients.

What You Can Do Now

- **Talk to your doctor early**: Before starting any new treatment, ask about how it may affect your fertility.
- **Get a referral**: You may need referral to a fertility specialist who works with patients to discuss options for preserving fertility in someone with chronic disease like lupus nephritis.
- **Keep lupus under control**: The best time to pursue pregnancy or fertility treatments is when your lupus is quiet or in remission for at least 6 months.
- **Discuss timing**: Pregnancy is safest when your lupus is stable, and kidney function is normal.

Many people with lupus nephritis go on to have children, even after treatment. With planning and teamwork between you, your nephrologist, rheumatologist, and a fertility expert, you can make choices that support your long-term health and enable a healthy and safe pregnancy.

Birth Control and Lupus Nephritis, What's Safe for You?

If you're living with lupus nephritis, choosing the right birth control is important. Not all methods are safe or ideal for everyone with lupus, especially if you have antiphospholipid antibodies or a history of blood clots. The right choice depends on your lupus activity, medications, kidney function, and personal preferences. Here we provide you with safe and effective contraception options and help you understand which methods to avoid.

Why Birth Control Matters

Even when you're not planning a pregnancy, having reliable birth control gives you control over your body and your health. This is especially important if:

- Your lupus is active or you're starting a new treatment.
- You're taking medications that are unsafe during pregnancy (like mycophenolate or methotrexate).
- You want to plan your pregnancy during a safe time, like when your lupus is in remission to enable having a safe and healthy pregnancy.

Important Factors to Consider

When choosing birth control, your doctor will consider:

- Lupus activity: Is your disease active or quiet (in remission)
- Antiphospholipid antibodies (aPL): These increase your risk for blood clots.
- History of blood clots or stroke
- Kidney function
- Current Medications
- Personal preference (daily pill vs long-term methods, hormonal vs non-hormonal)

Birth Control Options: What's Safe in Lupus Nephritis?

Birth Control Options for Women with Lupus (SLE)

Type of Birth Control	Safe if you don't have clotting antibodies	Safe if you do have clotting antibodies (aPL)	What to Know
Copper IUD (no hormones)	Yes	Yes	Very safe, lasts up to 10 years, no hormones
Hormonal IUD (e.g. Mirena)	Yes	Yes (ask your doctor)	Safe, releases a small amount of hormone in the uterus
Implant (in the arm, e.g. Nexplanon)	Yes	Yes (ask your doctor)	Long-lasting (3 years), very effective
Mini-pill (progestin-only pill)	Yes	Yes (ask your doctor)	Must take at the same time every day
Depo shot (injection every 3 months)	Yes (short-term)	Use with caution	Can lower bone strength, especially with steroid use
Pill/patch/ring with estrogen	Use with caution	No – not safe	Increases clot risk, avoid if you have clotting antibodies or a history of blood clots
Condoms or diaphragm	Yes	Yes	Safe but not the most reliable alone. Better when used with another method
Permanent options (tubal ligation or partner's vasectomy)	Yes	Yes	Good choice if you're sure you don't want kids in the future

Tips:

- Ask your doctor to test you for anti-Phospholipid antibodies (clotting antibodies) if you haven't been tested yet.
- Avoid estrogen-containing birth control if you have a history of blood clots or test positive for aPL.
- IUDs and implants are some of the safest and most effective options for people with lupus.
- If you take steroids, talk to your doctor before using the Depo shot due to bone health concerns.

What Should You Avoid?

Avoid birth control methods that contain estrogen if you have:

- Active lupus nephritis
- Positive antiphospholipid antibodies (aPL)
- History of deep vein thrombosis (DVT), stroke, or clotting problems

Estrogen-containing methods increase the risk of blood clots, which can be especially dangerous in lupus.

Your Next Steps

- Talk to your doctor or rheumatologist before starting or changing any birth control method.
- Ask whether you've been tested for aPL antibodies — this affects your options.
- If you're starting new medications for lupus nephritis, double-check whether pregnancy must be avoided (e.g., with mycophenolate).
- If you want to get pregnant in the future, discuss with your healthcare team about the safest time and medications for you and your baby during pregnancy.

You Deserve a Say in Your Reproductive Health

Choosing the right birth control means protecting your health and feeling in control. Whether you're planning or want to avoid unexpected risks now, there's a method that can work for you. You should discuss with your health care team.

Lupus Nephritis Medications — What's Safe During Pregnancy?

If you're pregnant or planning to become pregnant, it's natural to wonder how your medications might affect your baby. With lupus nephritis, staying on the right treatment is just as important as avoiding harmful drugs. We will discuss:

- Which medications are safe to take during pregnancy
- Which ones should be stopped or avoided
- How to plan pregnancy with your healthcare team

Why Medication Management Is So Important

Stopping lupus medications suddenly can be dangerous. Active lupus or lupus nephritis flares during pregnancy can harm both you and your baby — so it's often safer to adjust your medications rather than stop everything.

Work with your rheumatologist, nephrologist, and OB-GYN to find the right balance for both disease control and safe and healthy pregnancy.

Which Medications Are Safe?

Here's a table to help you understand which drugs are usually safe, need caution, or should be avoided in pregnancy:

Medication	Is It Safe During Pregnancy?	Comments
Hydroxychloroquine (Plaquenil)	Yes – *Strongly recommended*	Helps prevent flares; safe and protective during pregnancy.
Azathioprine (Imuran)	Yes (≤2 mg/kg/day)	Commonly used if immunosuppression is needed
Low-dose Aspirin	Yes (after 12 weeks)	Reduces risk of preeclampsia.
Tacrolimus (Prograf)	Yes (case-by-case)	Useful in flares; often used safely.
Cyclosporine	Yes (if needed)	Safe when benefits outweigh risks; used in resistant cases

Steroids (e.g., Prednisone)	Yes (use lowest effective dose)	Used to control flares. Higher doses carry some risk, but disease control is key
Methyldopa, Labetalol, Nifedipine	Yes	Safe options for treating high blood pressure
NSAIDs (e.g., ibuprofen)	Use with caution	Avoid after 20 weeks; never use after 30 weeks.

What Should Be Avoided?

Medication	**Why It's Unsafe**
Mycophenolate (Cellcept)	High risk of birth defects and miscarriage — stop at least 6 weeks before trying to conceive.
Methotrexate	Very harmful — must be stopped 6-12 weeks before pregnancy
Cyclophosphamide (Cytoxan)	Avoid in first trimester; only used in life-threatening cases later in pregnancy
Leflunomide	Possible birth defects — needs a special medication to wash it out before pregnancy
Voclosporin	Avoid — contains alcohol; risks to baby's development
Anifrolumab, SGLT2 inhibitors (dapagliflozin)	Not enough data — avoid during pregnancy and breastfeeding
Angiotensinogen convertase inhibitor/Angiotensin Receptor Blocker (lisinopril/losartan),	OK in first trimester but high risk of birth defects after that

Before You Get Pregnant: What to Ask

- Is this a safe for me to get pregnant?
- Are all my medications safe for pregnancy?
- Should I stop or switch anything before trying to conceive?

- Have I been off medications like mycophenolate or methotrexate long enough?
- Is my lupus nephritis quiet (in remission)?
- Is it possible for my lupus nephritis to flare during pregnancy?
- Do I need to adjust dose of medications before or during pregnancy?

During Pregnancy: Stay on Track

- Don't stop medications without medical advice.
- Keep your appointments with all specialists.
- If you're taking hydroxychloroquine or low-dose aspirin, don’t stop — they can help keep you and your baby safe.

Thinking About Pregnancy? Start with Pre-Pregnancy Counseling

If you have lupus nephritis and are thinking about having a baby, pre-pregnancy counseling is very important for you and your partner or family.

This is a special kind of doctor’s visit that helps you and your care team prepare for a safe and healthy pregnancy — for both you and your future baby.

Why Pre-Pregnancy Counseling Matters

Pregnancy with lupus nephritis is possible — but it does come with risks more than usual pregnancy. These risks are often much lower when:

- Your lupus and kidney disease are not active (in remission)
- You are on safe medications
- You are supported by a team of doctors who specialize in high-risk pregnancy

Pre-pregnancy counseling is where all of this begins.

When Should You Start Counseling?

Ideally, you should meet with your care team at least 6 months before trying to get pregnant. If that’s not possible, even a few months of preparation can make a difference.

What Happens at a Pre-Pregnancy Counseling Visit?

Your rheumatologist, nephrologist, and OB-GYN will work together to:

Review your medical history

They'll ask:

- When was your last lupus or kidney flare?
- Have you had any pregnancy complications in the past?
- Do you have any other health conditions (like high blood pressure or diabetes)?

Check your lupus activity

It's safest to get pregnant when your lupus has been quiet (in remission) for at least 6 months. Blood and urine tests can help confirm this.

Tests may include:

- Kidney function (creatinine)
- Urine protein levels
- Anti-dsDNA and complement (C3/C4) levels

Screen for high-risk factors

Certain antibodies like antiphospholipid (aPL) or anti-Ro/SSA and anti-La/SSB may raise your risk for pregnancy complications. Your doctor will test for these and discuss how to reduce the risks associated with them.

Review your medications

Some medications need to be stopped or changed before pregnancy like mycophenolate, methotrexate, or ACE inhibitors. Others medications like hydroxychloroquine should be continued.

You'll work together to adjust your treatment so it's both safe for pregnancy and effective for your lupus.

Discuss your goals and concerns

You'll have time to talk about:

- Your ideal timing for pregnancy

- Any past fertility issues
- Emotional readiness and support systems

What If My Lupus Isn't Fully Controlled Yet?

It's okay — many people with LN need to wait and stabilize before trying for pregnancy. Your doctor will help you get there safely, with regular check-ins and adjustments to your medications and care plan.

Your Health Comes First — So Your Pregnancy Can Too

Planning ahead gives you the best chance of a smooth pregnancy and a healthy baby. You deserve care that's not just safe, but thoughtful and empowering.

Managing Pregnancy with Lupus Nephritis — A Team Effort

Once you're pregnant, managing LN becomes a team effort. This journey isn't one you should walk alone, and you don't have to.

With the right support team, most women with LN can have a safe and healthy pregnancy.

Why Team-Based Care Matters

Pregnancy changes your body, and with lupus nephritis, those changes can sometimes be hard to tell apart from a flare. That's why it's essential to have multiple experts working together, all focused on you and your baby.

Who Should Be On Your Care Team?

Here are the key players:

Specialist	Role in Your Pregnancy
Nephrologist	Monitors kidney function, protein levels in urine, and manages blood pressure and LN flare
Rheumatologist	Oversees lupus activity and adjusts your medications
Maternal-Fetal Medicine OB (High-Risk OB)	Specializes in high-risk pregnancies like lupus and helps manage fetal monitoring and delivery planning

Primary OB/GYN	Provides general pregnancy care and coordinates with the high-risk OB
Pharmacist or Medication Safety Expert	Ensures all your medications are safe for pregnancy and breastfeeding
Nurse or Case Manager	Helps with scheduling, reminders, and emotional support.

What Does Pregnancy Management Look Like?

Your care team will:

- Monitor your lupus and kidneys every 4–6 weeks (or more often if needed)
- Check blood pressure, urine protein, and labs regularly
- Watch for signs of complications like preeclampsia or LN flares
- Perform frequent ultrasounds to track baby's growth
- Screen for congenital heart block if you're positive for anti-Ro/SSA or La/SSB antibodies
- Help plan timing and type of delivery

Communication Is Key

All your doctors should communicate regularly with each other. You can help by:

- Bringing updates between appointments
- Asking your providers to share notes and test results
- Keeping a list of your medications and symptoms
- Using a notebook or app to track questions and important info

What If There's a Flare or Complication?

Sometimes flares happen — even with good planning. If this occurs:

- Your team will adjust medications safely (e.g., steroids or pregnancy-safe immunosuppressants)
- In severe cases, hospital monitoring may be needed
- If delivery must happen early, a neonatal team will be ready to care for your baby

Remember: most flares can be managed without putting your baby at risk.

What Happens After Delivery?

You'll need close follow-up for at least 6 months postpartum:

- Lupus flares are more common after birth
- You may need medication changes if breastfeeding
- Your doctors will watch for blood clots, kidney flare, and mood changes

Your Role in the Team

You are the most important member of this team

Here's how you can stay involved:

- Ask questions and speak up about symptoms or concerns
- Take your medications as prescribed
- Keep all appointments, even when you feel well
- Make time for rest, hydration, nutrition, and emotional care

Pregnancy with lupus nephritis is complex, but you're not alone. With a strong care team and early planning, you can move through safe and healthy pregnancy with confidence and support — one step at a time.

Sources

- Sammaritano LR, Bermas BL, Chakravarty EE, Chambers C, Clowse MEB, Lockshin MD, et al. 2020 American College of Rheumatology Guideline for the Management of Reproductive Health in Rheumatic and Musculoskeletal Diseases. Arthritis Care Res (Hoboken). 2020;72(4):461–88. doi:10.1002/acr.24130
- Centers for Disease Control and Prevention. U.S. Medical Eligibility Criteria (MEC) for Contraceptive Use, 2020 Summary Chart. Atlanta, GA: CDC; 2020. Available from: https://www.cdc.gov/reproductivehealth/contraception/mmwr/mec/summary.html
- U.S. Food and Drug Administration. FDA Approves First Daily Oral Contraceptive for Over-the-Counter Use [Internet]. Silver Spring, MD: FDA; 2023 [cited 2025 May 20]. Available from:

https://www.fda.gov/news-events/press-announcements/fda-approves-first-daily-oral-contraceptive-over-counter-use

- Andreoli L, Bertsias GK, Agmon-Levin N, Brown S, Cervera R, Costedoat-Chalumeau N, et al. EULAR recommendations for women's health and the management of family planning, assisted reproduction, pregnancy and menopause in patients with systemic lupus erythematosus and/or antiphospholipid syndrome. Ann Rheum Dis. 2017;76(3):476–85. doi:10.1136/annrheumdis-2016-209770
- National Institutes of Health (NIH). Contraception for Women with Lupus [Internet]. Bethesda, MD: NIH; 2023 [cited 2025 May 20]. Available from: https://www.nichd.nih.gov/health/topics/lupus/conditioninfo/treatment#contraception
- Gholizadeh Ghozloujeh Z, Singh T, Jhaveri KD, Shah S, Lerma E, Abdipour A and Norouzi S (2024) Lupus nephritis: management challenges during pregnancy. *Front. Nephrol.* 4:1390783. doi: 10.3389/fneph.2024.1390783

CHAPTER 9

MANAGING THE COSTS OF CARE

FIND WAYS TO EASE FINANCIAL STRESS OF TREATMENT

Abstract

This chapter explores the profound financial burden of lupus nephritis through the lens of a hypothetical patient, Mia. It highlights how the high cost of medications, hospitalizations, specialist visits, and diagnostic tests can destabilize families, even for those with insurance. Beyond direct costs, the chapter addresses lost wages, transportation expenses, and the mental toll of chronic financial stress. It emphasizes the need for systemic solutions, including better insurance coverage, access to generics, patient assistance programs, and employer flexibility. By detailing the economic challenges, the chapter calls for a more compassionate, equitable healthcare system for those with lupus nephritis.

Keywords: Lupus Nephritis, Financial Burden, Medication Costs, Healthcare Access, Patient Assistance Programs

Let's start this chapter with Mia's hypothetical story. The burden of illness is often felt most acutely in the quiet moments when the relentless pace of life slows down and reality seeps in like the cold of a winter's night. For Mia, a 34-year-old single mother, the weight of her lupus nephritis diagnosis was not just a personal struggle; it was a looming shadow over her family's financial stability.

Mia had always been the pillar of strength for her two young children, juggling a part-time job while managing their daily needs. After years of enduring unexplained fatigue, joint pain, and frequent hospital visits, her doctor finally delivered the diagnosis that would change everything—Lupus nephritis. The words echoed in her mind, carrying with them a sense of dread about her health and the uncertain future ahead.

As she sat at the kitchen table, bills scattered around her like fallen leaves, the reality of her situation began to sink in. The cost of medications, specialist visits, and necessary treatments was staggering. Even with insurance, the out-of-pocket expenses seemed insurmountable. Mia found herself caught in a cycle of anxiety, constantly calculating how to make ends meet while ensuring her children's needs were met.

Every month brought new challenges. There were days when she had to choose between her medication and groceries, each decision filled with guilt and despair. She could see the worry etched on her children's faces, innocent eyes trying to comprehend why their mother was often too tired to play or stressed to engage in their lives fully. Mia's thoughts spiraled: What would happen if her condition worsened? Would she be able to keep her job? How would they survive?

Mia's journey through lupus nephritis illuminated a harsh reality faced by many patients: the financial burden of chronic illness extends far beyond medical costs. It infiltrates families, disrupts livelihoods, and can leave lasting scars on mental health. As she navigated her new reality, Mia knew she wasn't alone. Many others shared her plight, trapped in a system that often prioritized profit over patient care, struggling with the devastating financial implications of their health conditions.

This chapter explores the complex costs of lupus nephritis, highlighting the direct and indirect financial effects on patients such as Mia. We hope to illuminate the genuine expenses of managing this chronic condition and promote a healthcare system that values patient well-being over profit.

Cost of living with lupus and lupus nephritis

Managing patients with lupus creates a significant financial burden on the healthcare system. This means that treating people with lupus costs a lot of money, both for patients and for the healthcare system. Studies have shown that the average annual costs related to lupus can vary widely. Direct costs, which include medical care and medications, range from about $2,214 to $16,875 per year. Indirect costs, including lost wages when patients can't work, can range from $2,239 to $35,540 annually (1, 2).

Medications make up a substantial part of the total costs for patients with lupus, accounting for about 19% to 30% of their spending. Regarding other medical expenses, costs for hospital stays (inpatient care) and visits to the doctor (outpatient care) are also high. Inpatient care, i.e., hospitalization costs, can make up 16% to 50% of total expenses, while outpatient care can account for 24% to 56% of overall costs (1, 2).

However, the financial impact is even more significant for patients with lupus nephritis. The average direct costs for these patients can range from $29,034 to $62,651 each year. This shows lupus nephritis is expensive compared to other forms of lupus (1, 3).

Additionally, as the disease progresses or leads to increased organ damage, expenses often escalate further. This implies that individuals experiencing severe symptoms or complications will encounter higher financial strains due to treatment costs and possibly inability to work due to disease activity. Sadly, despite the considerable costs linked to lupus nephritis, there has been limited research focused on the economic challenges that the patients endure. More studies are needed to understand the impact of chronic diseases like Lupus Nephritis and discover methods to alleviate these costs for patients and the healthcare system (4-6).

The High Cost of Long-Term Treatment for Lupus Nephritis

Living with lupus nephritis can be quite challenging physically, mentally, and financially. This condition impacts the kidneys and is a significant complication of lupus, an autoimmune disease. Managing lupus nephritis typically involves ongoing treatment that can come with a hefty price tag. Patients and their families need to be aware of these costs.

A. Medication Costs:

One of the most considerable costs for individuals with lupus nephritis is the price of medications. These treatments are essential as they assist in managing the condition and safeguarding the kidneys from harm. Let's take a closer look at the various types of medications typically used and their associated costs:

1. Immunosuppressants: These medications help to calm the immune system, which is important since lupus can lead the body to unintentionally harm its kidneys. Some examples of these drugs are mycophenolate mofetil and azathioprine. However, without insurance, the monthly costs for these medications can reach the hundreds of dollars. This can create a considerable financial strain for patients, particularly for those already facing other expenses related to their condition.

2. Corticosteroids: These medications are often used to reduce inflammation and manage symptoms. They can be very effective in quickly improving a patient's condition. However, using corticosteroids for a long time can lead to side effects, such as weight gain, mood swings, and increased risk of infections. While they may help in the short term, the long-term effects and the need for additional medications to counteract these side effects can add to the overall treatment costs.

3. Biologics: Newer medications target specific parts of the immune system. One example is belimumab, which is very effective for some patients. However, biologics can be expensive, sometimes costing thousands of dollars yearly. The high cost of these medications can make it difficult for patients to afford them, even with insurance (7, 8).

Many patients find themselves stressed about how to pay for these medications. Even if they have insurance, the out-of-pocket costs can be significant. Patients may face high deductibles or copays, meaning they must pay a portion of the cost themselves. This financial pressure can lead to difficult choices, such as paying for necessary medications and covering other essential expenses, like groceries or rent.

Additionally, some patients may experience delays in starting or continuing their medications due to the costs. In the long run, this can worsen health, cause more frequent hospital visits, and even cause higher overall costs. The cycle of needing treatment but being unable to afford it is a harsh reality for many living with lupus nephritis.

B. Doctor Visits and Tests:

In addition to medications, patients with lupus nephritis must visit their doctors regularly. These visits are crucial for monitoring their health and ensuring the treatment works effectively. Regular check-ups allow healthcare providers to assess kidney function, adjust medications as necessary, and monitor for any side effects of medications.

However, each visit to the doctor can come with additional costs that patients need to consider. Here are some common expenses associated with doctor visits:

1. Copays: A copay is a fixed amount that patients pay for each doctor visit. This amount can vary widely depending on the insurance plan. For example, a patient may have to pay $20 for a visit, while another may face a $50 copay. Over time, these costs can add up, especially for patients who need to see their doctors frequently.

2. Transportation Costs: Traveling to and from medical appointments can also become a financial burden. Patients may need to visit multiple specialists, such as nephrologists, rheumatologists, and primary care doctors. If they rely on public transportation, the costs can add up quickly. For those who drive, expenses like gas, parking fees, and wear-and-tear on their vehicles can further strain their budgets.

3. Testing Expenses: Patients often need blood tests, urine tests, and other diagnostic procedures to monitor how well their kidneys are functioning. These tests are essential for understanding the disease's progression and making treatment decisions. Even though some tests may be covered by insurance, patients can still face out-of-pocket expenses. For example, if a patient has a high deductible insurance plan, they might have to pay for the total cost of tests until they meet their deductible. The costs for tests can vary, but they often range from $100 to several hundred dollars, depending on the type of test performed.

4. Loss of work: Patients with Lupus Nephritis have at least three specialists, rheumatologists, nephrologists, and ophthalmologists, along with their primary care doctor visits. All specialists need their tests done before their clinic visit. All the clinic visits and time needed to do lab tests increase over time. Some people do not get paid time off, and they have to consider lost pay to make to the doctor's visit.

Research shows that the average annual healthcare costs for patients with lupus nephritis are significantly higher compared to those without the disease (9, 10). This expense increase can be attributed to the need for regular doctor visits, specialized care, and ongoing monitoring through various tests.

All these factors together make managing lupus nephritis quite costly. Patients are frequently concerned about their health and how to afford the essential care they need.

C. Hospitalizations:

Sometimes, patients with lupus nephritis experience severe flares of the disease, which can require hospitalization. A flare is when the disease becomes more active, leading to increased symptoms and complications.

Patients may need intensive medical care to manage their condition and protect their kidneys during these times.

Several studies have shown that patients with lupus nephritis experience higher annual healthcare costs compared to those with lupus who do not have nephritis. This notable expense rise is mainly attributed to inpatient admissions, pharmacy services, and outpatient care (11, 12). Another study found that about 25% of patients with LN experienced at least one hospitalization within the year following their diagnosis, with the average total healthcare costs per patient annually amounting to $45,469 (13).

If a patient must be hospitalized several times a year due to recurring flares, the medical bills can add up. Many families struggle with these high costs, especially when they're already managing the expenses of medications and regular doctor visits.

The anxiety about potential medical bills can be quite overwhelming for many patients. This financial worry can create a cycle of fear that impacts their overall health and well-being. Some patients might even hesitate to seek hospital care when it's truly necessary, concerned about the costs that may follow. Unfortunately, delaying treatment can worsen their condition and lead to even higher medical expenses. Patients must remember that taking care of their health should be a priority, even amidst financial worries.

Managing lupus nephritis is challenging enough without the added pressure of financial concerns. By staying informed and reaching out for help when needed, patients can better navigate the complexities of their care and focus on what truly matters: their health.

In summary, managing lupus and nephritis can financially challenge patients and the healthcare system. The annual direct costs for lupus can vary significantly, and when you factor in indirect costs, the overall expenses can add up. For those dealing with lupus nephritis, the financial impact is even more pronounced, as the costs of managing their condition can be quite substantial. Many of these expenses come from medications, hospital stays, and outpatient care, contributing to medical bills. Patients often encounter various costs, such as copays for doctor visits, transportation for medical appointments, and necessary tests. This financial pressure can lead to anxiety, causing some patients to hesitate in seeking the hospital care they need due to worries about high bills, which can ultimately affect their health. Patients need to focus on their health while also navigating these financial hurdles.

The need for support

Living with lupus nephritis can bring about various challenges that may significantly affect patients' physical health, emotional well-being, and financial stability. To truly support these individuals, it's important to implement thorough strategies that cater to their unique needs. Here are some potential solutions that can offer valuable assistance:

- **Better Insurance Coverage:** Enhancing insurance plans can significantly lighten the financial load for patients. This means expanding the range of covered medications and ensuring that crucial doctor visits and diagnostic tests are part of the coverage. Policies could be tailored to remove high deductibles or copays for essential treatments, making healthcare more accessible. Furthermore, encouraging insurance companies to embrace value-based care models—where reimbursement is tied to patient outcomes rather than the number of services provided—could improve patient support and management.
  It is beneficial to meet with a healthcare insurance specialist either at your workplace or at the hospital system where you get your medical care to discuss which would be the best insurance plan for you and your family's needs.
- **Access to Generic Medications:** Access to generic medications can significantly reduce treatment expenses for patients with lupus nephritis. These generics are frequently just as effective as their brand-name counterparts but come at a much lower cost. To support this, healthcare providers can be trained to discuss generic options with their patients and promote their use when suitable. Policymakers can also help by simplifying the approval process for generics, making sure they become available on the market swiftly and safely. Furthermore, informing patients about the effectiveness of generics can help alleviate any concerns they might have about using them.
- **Patient Assistance Programs:** Numerous pharmaceutical companies understand the financial strain medications can impose on patients, so they've created patient assistance programs. These programs can differ significantly, providing everything from discounts to free medications depending on one's income and needs. It's important for

healthcare providers to share this information with patients and for patients to inquire about these options proactively. Healthcare professionals can offer valuable advice on applying for these programs and assist patients in navigating the application process.

- **Education and Resources:** It's imperative to offer thorough education about lupus nephritis and how to manage it. This can be done through workshops, printed guides, online resources, and community outreach initiatives. Educational sessions can touch on understanding the disease, spotting symptoms, managing medications, and planning for healthcare costs. Resources that assist patients in learning about financial planning and dealing with insurance can also help them make informed choices. Additionally, providing training for healthcare providers on the unique challenges faced by lupus nephritis patients can enhance the support they offer.
- **Support Networks:** Building strong support networks can significantly improve the emotional health of patients. Support groups, whether face-to-face or online, allow patients to connect with others with similar experiences. These groups can provide emotional backing, practical tips, and a sense of belonging. Plus, having access to mental health professionals who focus on chronic illnesses can assist patients in managing feelings of anxiety, depression, and isolation that frequently come with their diagnosis. Nurturing an environment where patients feel safe to share their challenges can encourage resilience and hope.
- **Navigating Employment Challenges:** Many patients with lupus nephritis face difficulties maintaining their employment due to the unpredictable nature of their symptoms. Employers can play a crucial role by offering flexible work arrangements, such as telecommuting options or modified schedules. Organizations should also be encouraged to educate themselves about lupus and its impact on employees. Disability benefits and workplace accommodations are essential in supporting patients professionally while managing their health.
- **Advocacy and Policy Change:** Advocating at the community and national levels can bring about meaningful changes that positively impact patients with lupus nephritis. By supporting policies that enhance healthcare access, make medications more affordable, and ensure comprehensive insurance coverage, we can help create a fairer system. Grassroots efforts and partnerships with healthcare organizations can increase awareness of lupus nephritis, fostering initiatives that cater to the unique needs of these patients.

Conclusion

In summary, offering strong support for patients with lupus nephritis is vital for enhancing their quality of life and health results. By improving insurance coverage, expanding access to generic medications, providing patient assistance programs, educating patients, building support networks, tackling employment issues, and advocating for policy changes, we can help ease the challenges of this chronic condition. These efforts not only empower patients to manage their health effectively but also foster a fairer and more supportive healthcare system that puts the needs of all patients first.

Take home points

- Managing lupus and lupus nephritis creates a significant financial burden on patients and the healthcare system.
- Medications constitute a significant expense for lupus patients, alongside costs from hospitalizations and doctor visits.
- As lupus progresses and causes more organ damage, the financial strain on patients increases substantially.
- Financial anxiety can discourage patients from seeking necessary medical care, jeopardizing their health further.
- Comprehensive support strategies are essential to alleviate the challenges faced by patients, including better insurance, access to generics and educational resources

References

1. Slawsky KA, Fernandes AW, Fusfeld L, Manzi S, Goss TF. A structured literature review of the direct costs of adult systemic lupus erythematosus in the US. Arthritis Care Res (Hoboken). 2011;63(9):1224-32.
2. Meacock R, Dale N, Harrison MJ. The humanistic and economic burden of systemic lupus erythematosus : a systematic review. Pharmacoeconomics. 2013;31(1):49-61.
3. Turchetti G, Yazdany J, Palla I, Yelin E, Mosca M. Systemic lupus erythematosus and the economic perspective: a systematic literature review and points to consider. Clin Exp Rheumatol. 2012;30(4 Suppl 73):S116-22.

4. Zhu TY, Tam LS, Lee VW, Lee KK, Li EK. The impact of flare on disease costs of patients with systemic lupus erythematosus. Arthritis Rheum. 2009;61(9):1159-67.
5. Panopalis P, Petri M, Manzi S, Isenberg DA, Gordon C, Senecal JL, et al. The systemic lupus erythematosus Tri-Nation study: cumulative indirect costs. Arthritis Rheum. 2007;57(1):64-70.
6. Kan H, Guerin A, Kaminsky MS, Yu AP, Wu EQ, Denio A, et al. A longitudinal analysis of costs associated with change in disease activity in systemic lupus erythematosus. J Med Econ. 2013;16(6): 793-800.
7. Petrou P. A Systematic Review of the Economic Evaluations of Belimumab in Systemic Lupus Erythematosus. Value Health Reg Issues. 2022;27:32-40.
8. Alsuwayegh A, Almaghlouth IA, Almasaoud MA, Alzaid AS, Alsuhaibani AA, Almana LH, et al. Cost Consequence Analysis of Belimumab versus Standard of Care for the Management of Systemic Lupus Erythematosus in Saudi Arabia: A Retrospective Cohort Study. Int J Environ Res Public Health. 2023;20(3).
9. Thompson JC, Mahajan A, Scott DA, Gairy K. The Economic Burden of Lupus Nephritis: A Systematic Literature Review. Rheumatol Ther. 2022;9(1):25-47.
10. Bell CF, Wu B, Huang SP, Rubin B, Averell CM, Chastek B, et al. Healthcare resource utilization and costs in patients with a newly confirmed diagnosis of lupus nephritis in the United States over a 5-year follow-up period. BMC Health Serv Res. 2024;24(1):691.
11. Pelletier EM, Ogale S, Yu E, Brunetta P, Garg J. Economic outcomes in patients diagnosed with systemic lupus erythematosus with versus without nephritis: results from an analysis of data from a US claims database. Clin Ther. 2009;31(11):2653-64.
12. Li T, Carls GS, Panopalis P, Wang S, Gibson TB, Goetzel RZ. Long-term medical costs and resource utilization in systemic lupus erythematosus and lupus nephritis: a five-year analysis of a large medicaid population. Arthritis Rheum. 2009;61(6):755-63.
13. Bartels-Peculis L, Sharma A, Edwards AM, Sanyal A, Connolly-Strong E, Nelson WW. Treatment Patterns and Health Care Costs of Lupus Nephritis in a United States Payer Population. Open Access Rheumatol. 2020;12:117-24.

CHAPTER 10

LIFE AFTER KIDNEY TRANSPLANT

DISCOVER NEW POSSIBILITIES FOR HEALTH AND LIVING

Abstract

This chapter explores kidney transplantation as a vital option for patients with lupus nephritis who progress to end-stage kidney disease. Through Lily's narrative, it illustrates the emotional and clinical journey of preparing for and recovering from a transplant. It addresses when to consider transplant, the effects of lupus activity in dialysis patients, transplant timing, donor options, and immunosuppressive strategies. The chapter also examines the recurrence risks of lupus nephritis in transplanted kidneys, especially among high-risk populations. Emphasizing personalized care and vigilant monitoring underscores transplantation's potential to significantly enhance the quality of life in lupus nephritis.

Keywords: Lupus Nephritis, Kidney Transplantation, End-Stage Kidney Disease (ESKD), Immunosuppression, Recurrence Risk

Let's start this chapter with Lily's hypothetical case. Lily, a lively 28-year-old, has always approached life with boundless enthusiasm. As a graphic designer, she channels her creativity into every project, often losing herself in her work. However, about a year ago, she started facing some challenges that dimmed her bright spirit—constant fatigue, joint pain that turned even the simplest tasks into significant hurdles, and a distinctive butterfly rash that appeared on her cheeks. Following numerous tests, she received a diagnosis that transformed her life: systemic lupus erythematosus.

At first, Lily faced her diagnosis with a positive attitude. With a wealth of information and a solid support network, she effectively managed her condition through medication, consistent doctor visits, and lifestyle changes. However, as time went by, her health began to decline. During a routine check-up, her nephrologist, Dr. Patel, shared some tough news: her lupus had advanced to lupus nephritis, causing considerable damage to her kidneys.

Even though Lily followed her treatment plan closely, her kidney function continued to decline, and she eventually had to confront the reality of end-stage renal disease (ESRD). The thought of starting dialysis weighed heavily on her, dimming her previously optimistic outlook. During a heartfelt discussion with Dr. Patel, she discovered her options: she could stay on dialysis right away or explore kidney transplantation as a more hopeful choice.

Facing an uncertain future, Lily decided to go for a kidney transplant. The idea of regaining her life without the constraints of dialysis sparked a glimmer of hope in her heart. With the unwavering support of her family and friends, she embarked on the intricate journey of the transplant process.

The pre-transplant evaluation was quite a journey for Lily. She underwent extensive medical assessments, psychological evaluations, and several compatibility tests. Each step brought a mix of hope and nervousness as she navigated the complex world of waiting lists and potential donors. Throughout this process, she leaned heavily on her loved ones, finding comfort in their unwavering support.

One day, while Lily anxiously awaited her evaluation results, she found herself in a bustling hospital waiting room surrounded by patients, each on their unique journeys. She began chatting with a kind older woman named Margaret, who had triumphantly undergone a kidney transplant a year earlier. Margaret generously shared her experiences with Lily, providing comforting advice and encouragement. “It’s a challenging path, but there’s light at the end. Just hold on to the belief that you’ll make it,” she said, her face lighting up with a warm smile.

Eventually, the day came when Lily received the call she had been waiting for. A suitable donor had been found, and she was scheduled for surgery. As she prepared for the transplant, she reflected on her journey, feeling a blend of fear and exhilaration. The surgery was a success, and Lily woke up post-op surrounded by her family, who were eager to celebrate this new beginning with her.

Lily’s recovery journey was not without its challenges. She faced the ongoing management of her lupus, the adjustment to a new regimen of immunosuppressive medications, and the need for constant monitoring to ensure her body accepted the new kidney. But she embraced these challenges, motivated by the vision of a life unbound by dialysis.

Lily's journey is a beautiful example of resilience, hope, and how kidney transplantation can change lives for those battling lupus nephritis. As we explore the details of this process in this chapter, Lily's story will highlight the significant effects such a transformative decision can have on individuals and their families and communities.

When to consider Kidney transplantation in patients with lupus nephritis

The primary objective in treating lupus nephritis is to delay the progression of kidney damage. Despite medical interventions, some patients may experience an ongoing decline in kidney function. Here are some essential scenarios when patients with lupus nephritis are recommended for a kidney transplant:

1. Progressive decline in kidney function:

Nephrologists caring for patients with Lupus Nephritis prioritize monitoring their kidney function closely. This entails regular testing of key parameters like the glomerular filtration rate (GFR), which assesses the kidneys' waste-filtering efficiency. A GFR drop to 20 ml/min/1.73 m^2 or below indicates a significant decline in kidney function, suggesting they struggle to perform essential tasks. At this stage, a kidney transplant referral is typically initiated to assess and prepare the patient for transplantation before dialysis becomes necessary. This proactive strategy facilitates a smoother transition and potentially improves patient outcomes.

Recommending a kidney transplant before the need for dialysis helps preserve the patient's quality of life and overall health. Anticipating the need for a transplant and starting the referral process early can offer a window of opportunity for patients to receive a new kidney while they are still relatively healthy. This strategy helps avoid complications and lifestyle disruptions associated with dialysis, improving the chances of a successful transplant and better post-operative recovery.

2. End-stage kidney disease:

If kidney function continues to decline in individuals with Lupus Nephritis and the kidneys cannot effectively filter waste from the blood, it may be necessary to initiate dialysis. This typically happens when Lupus Nephritis advances to end-stage kidney disease when a significant loss of kidney function has happened. Persistent kidney failure is indicated by elevated levels of waste products in the blood, uncontrolled blood pressure, and substantial protein loss in the urine. These signs imply that the kidneys are no longer capable of supporting essential bodily functions, resulting in the accumulation of harmful substances that may impact overall health and quality of life.

When patients with Lupus Nephritis require dialysis, it underscores the severity of their condition and the need for more intensive management strategies. Dialysis helps to perform the essential functions of the kidneys by removing waste products and excess fluids from the blood, but it is not a cure.

For these patients, a referral for kidney transplant evaluation becomes crucial. A kidney transplant can help bring back normal kidney function, improving the patient's quality of life and minimizing the long-term health issues that can come with dialysis. The transplant evaluation process includes assessing the patient's overall health, compatibility with a donor kidney, and readiness for surgery and post-operative care. By considering a kidney transplant, patients and their healthcare teams can work towards a more sustainable and effective treatment plan for managing advanced Lupus Nephritis.

Exploring Lupus Activity in Patients with End-Stage Kidney Disease

When patients with lupus nephritis reach end-stage kidney disease and start dialysis, it's common to see a significant decrease in both the clinical and serological activity of lupus. This has been widely observed in both clinical settings and research, showing that those facing kidney failure from lupus often experience a remission of lupus symptoms that goes beyond just the kidneys. For many, starting dialysis significantly improves lupus-related lab results, indicating that end-stage kidney disease is an immunosuppressive state. Some patients may find that they no longer need immunosuppressive medications to control their lupus symptoms. Numerous studies have highlighted these improvements in various autoimmune symptoms after beginning dialysis, suggesting that kidney failure may unexpectedly lessen the systemic effects of lupus (1-4).

The exact mechanisms behind this reduction in lupus activity following the start of dialysis remain unclear, yet the trend is consistently noted in various patient populations. Many individuals report a gradual or partial improvement in symptoms affecting different body systems after beginning dialysis treatment. This observation has led to the belief that the dialysis process might play a role in removing circulating autoantibodies or inflammatory mediators contributing to lupus pathology. Furthermore, restoring fluid and electrolyte balance homeostasis during dialysis may also positively impact overall immune function, thus alleviating some of the systemic symptoms associated with lupus.

However, it is essential to recognize that this pattern of improvement is not universal. Certain patients, especially those with severe disease, may still experience persistent lupus activity or a worsening of symptoms upon reaching end-stage kidney disease. These cases, although less frequent, highlight the importance of individualized care and close supervision for all lupus patients undergoing dialysis. The variability in responses underscores the necessity for nephrologists and healthcare providers to tailor treatment plans according to each patient's unique needs, considering genetic, environmental, and disease-specific factors that may influence lupus activity during dialysis (5, 6).

In short, although many patients with lupus nephritis experience notable improvements after starting dialysis, some may still struggle with their lupus symptoms. Continued research is essential to uncover the underlying mechanisms and create strategies to enhance care for all lupus nephritis patients, especially those moving to dialysis. As we progress in this field, incorporating personalized medicine and diligent monitoring will be key to improving outcomes for this varied group of patients.

Timing of transplantation in patients with lupus nephritis

When considering kidney transplantation for patients diagnosed with end-stage kidney disease, there are no universally established guidelines dictating the precise timing for the procedure. Each patient's situation is unique, and medical professionals typically evaluate various factors before recommending transplantation.

In general, it is advisable to proceed with a kidney transplant when the lupus is in a stable state and not currently active. This recommendation stems from the understanding that active autoimmune diseases, like lupus, may increase the risks associated with surgery and post-operative recovery and potentially complicate the long-term management of the transplanted kidney (7-9).

Interestingly, research has shown that the level of disease activity at the time of transplantation does not significantly influence the overall success rates of the transplant. This suggests that while it is preferable for lupus to be inactive during the kidney transplant procedure, patients with varying disease activity levels can still achieve favorable outcomes following a kidney transplant (10, 11).

Ultimately, the decision regarding the timing of the transplant should be made collaboratively by the patient and their healthcare team, considering the patient's overall health, the status of their kidney disease, the activity of any underlying conditions, and the potential risks and benefits associated with the procedure. Regular monitoring and a tailored approach to each patient's care are essential in ensuring the best possible outcomes.

Kidney transplant options

Patients with end-stage kidney disease or advanced chronic kidney disease from lupus nephritis have multiple kidney transplant options (figure 1).

Figure 1: Options for a kidney transplant.

A. A. Living donor kidney transplant:

Choosing a living donor kidney transplant is a fantastic option for two key reasons:

- Patients can receive a kidney without waiting on the transplant list.
- Kidneys from living donors tend to have a significantly longer lifespan and continue to function effectively for a longer time.

B. Deceased donor kidney transplants:

The kidneys from deceased donors are obtained after the donor has passed away. There are two main drawbacks to kidney transplants from deceased donors:

- Recipients often face longer waiting times for a kidney allograft, which varies by blood group—those with blood group O typically wait the longest, while those with blood group A have shorter wait times.

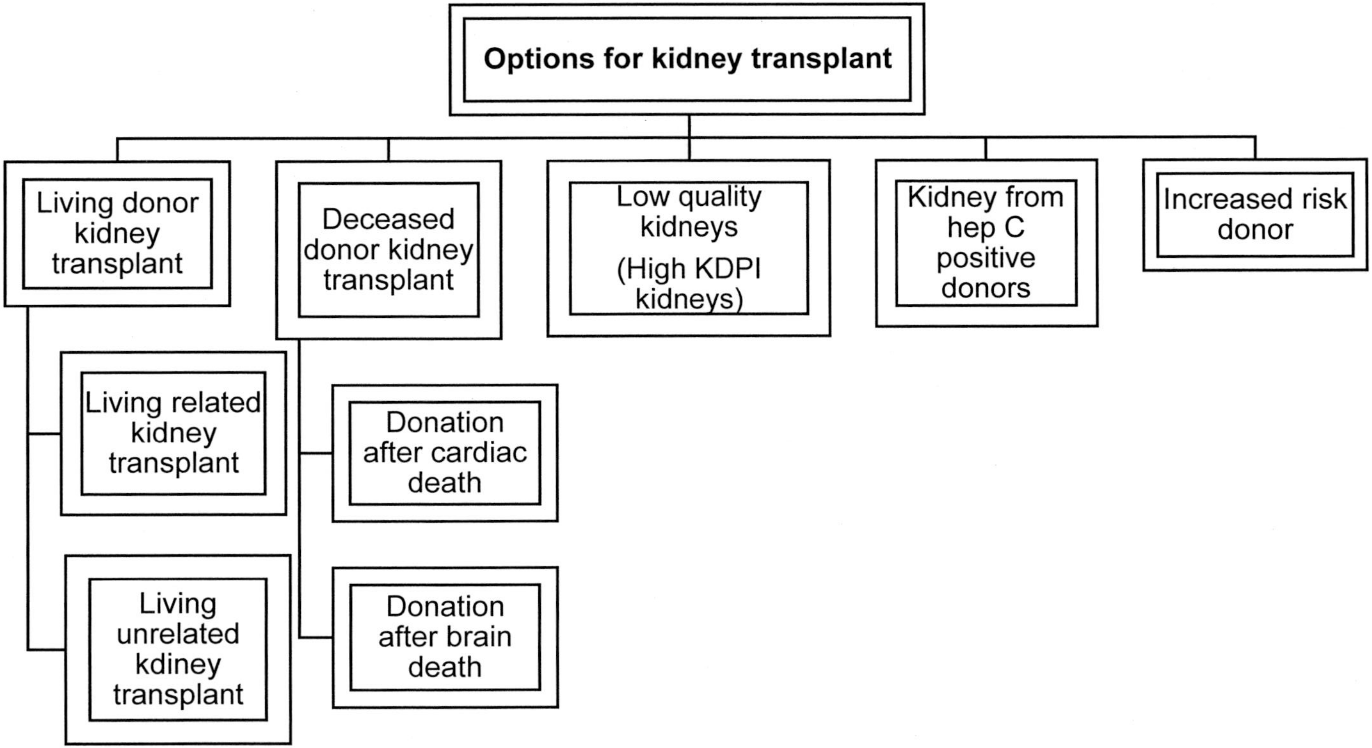
Options for kidney transplant
Living donor kidney transplant
Deceased donor kidney transplant
Low quality kidneys (High KDPI kidneys)
Kidney from hep C positive donors
Increased risk donor
Living related kidney transplant
Living unrelated kdiney transplant
Donation after cardiac death
Donation after brain death

- Additionally, kidneys from deceased donors tend to have a shorter half-life than those from living donors.

C. Low-quality kidneys (Donors with Kidney profile Index – KDPI > 85%):

KDPI is derived from the multiple factors as given in Table 1.

Table 1: Factor determines the KDPI score.

Factors – which determine the KDPI
1. Age
2. Height
3. Weight
4. Race
5. Diabetes
6. Hypertension
7. Cause of death – Stroke, cardiac death, motor vehicle accident, etc.
8. Serum creatinine
9. Hepatitis C status

The KDPI score helps us understand how likely a kidney transplant will succeed after the procedure. A lower KDPI score means the kidney is expected to function longer, while a higher score suggests a shorter lifespan for the transplant.

If a kidney has a KDPI greater than 85%, special consent is required to use it. Generally, high KDPI kidneys are not advised for younger patients who are healthy, without diabetes, and don't have significant heart issues. Instead, these kidneys are typically recommended for older patients who may have diabetes or significant heart conditions and have been waiting a long time for a transplant.

D. Kidneys from hepatitis C positive donor:

Hepatitis is a viral infection that impacts the liver, and hepatitis C primarily spreads through blood. In the past, kidneys from hepatitis C-infected donors were often discarded. However, thanks to the advancements in hepatitis C treatments over the last ten years, these kidneys can now be utilized for patients requiring a kidney transplant. There's over a 90% likelihood that recipients of these kidneys will contract hepatitis C, but the good news is that they can be effectively treated within a few months after the transplant.

Table 2: Advantages and disadvantages of kidneys from hepatitis C-positive donors.

Kidneys from the hepatitis C-positive donor	
Advantages	**Disadvantages**
Reduce time on the waitlist	More than 90% risk of getting hepatitis C; however, it can be treated effectively for a few months post-transplant
Kidney quality kidneys	

E. Increased risk donors:

High-risk donors are defined by certain donor characteristics described in Table 3.

Table 3: Characteristics of the high-risk donors

Characteristics of the high-risk donors:
1. People who had sex with a person known or suspected to have HIV or hepatitis B or C in the last 12 months
2. Men who had sex with other men in the previous 12 months and women who had sex with one of these men
3. People who have had sex in exchange for drugs or money and anyone who has sex with one of these individuals
4. People who have abused IV drugs or have had sex with someone who has used IV drugs in the last one year
5. People who have been in jail for more than 72 hours in the previous 12 months
6. People who have had multiple drug transfusions
7. People whose medical and social history cannot be obtained

Before the transplant, every organ undergoes a comprehensive assessment to minimize the risk of transmission. The chance of disease transmission through an organ transplant is very low.

The recipient is always notified if a donor is classified as a "high-risk" donor. Recipients can decline the high-risk kidney without affecting their position on the waiting list.

Advantages of kidney transplantation

Kidney transplantation has several advantages over dialysis. These advantages are described in Table 4.

Table 4: Advantages of kidney transplantation

Advantages of kidney transplantation
1. Improved mortality (Increased lifespan as compared to being on dialysis)
2. Improved quality of life
3. Can go back to work like anyone who has no kidney problem
4. No specific dietary restrictions that patients have to follow while on dialysis

Immunosuppression consideration for patients with lupus nephritis

For patients with lupus nephritis who receive a kidney transplant, it's crucial to take certain medications called immunosuppressants for their health and recovery. These medications are key in stopping the body from rejecting the new kidney. Because lupus nephritis can impact both the kidneys and other organs, using immunosuppressants is also essential to help avoid a return of lupus symptoms in the transplanted kidney. This thoughtful approach helps ensure the new kidney works effectively and supports the patient's health.

While immunosuppressants are essential, it is important to recognize that some medications commonly used to treat lupus nephritis, such as cyclophosphamide and mycophenolate, come with potential risks. These drugs can increase the likelihood of bone marrow suppression, which may lead to decreased production of blood cells. This condition can make patients more vulnerable to infections, anemia, and other complications. Additionally, long-term use of certain immunosuppressants is associated with a higher risk of developing certain types of cancers. Therefore, healthcare providers must carefully select the most appropriate immunosuppressive medications tailored to each patient's unique needs, balancing the benefits of preventing rejection with the potential risks involved.

After the kidney transplant, ongoing monitoring is crucial. Doctors will closely observe patients for any signs of infection or abnormalities that could indicate a return of lupus activity or cancer development. Regular check-ups and lab tests are essential to assess kidney function and to monitor blood cell counts, ensuring that any issues are detected early and managed promptly. This vigilant approach helps safeguard the patient's health and improves their chances of long-term success after transplantation.

Furthermore, patient education plays an essential role in this process. Patients should be informed about the importance of adhering to their medication regimen, recognizing symptoms that may indicate complications, and maintaining regular follow-up appointments. Empowering patients with knowledge about their condition and treatment can lead to better health outcomes and a smoother transition into life after kidney transplantation.

Recurrent lupus nephritis after kidney transplant

Lupus nephritis, along with other kidney diseases, has the potential to return in a transplanted kidney. This can be a concern for individuals with lupus who have undergone a kidney transplant. Lupus nephritis in the new kidney can vary greatly, with rates reported between 0% and 54% (12-16). It is essential to be aware that while some patients may not experience a recurrence, others may encounter this issue. The chance of recurrence is a crucial factor to consider for patients and their healthcare providers when discussing a kidney transplant. Being informed about this risk is valuable for decision-making and preparing for potential outcomes. Thanks to modern immunosuppression medications, the chance of lupus nephritis coming back has significantly decreased (17).

When lupus nephritis reoccurs in a transplanted kidney, it can lead to various issues affecting the kidney's function. Patients may notice a sudden rise in serum creatinine levels, indicating the kidney's efficiency in filtering waste. This could signal that the kidney is not functioning optimally. Other signs of recurring lupus nephritis include a gradual increase in creatinine levels from the baseline, hinting at a slow decline in kidney function. Patients might also observe new protein in the urine, which is abnormal and suggests kidney damage. Blood in the urine could be another indicator, sometimes with protein and blood present.

Managing the recurrence of lupus nephritis in a transplanted kidney can be challenging, but early detection and treatment are crucial. Patients should stay vigilant for symptoms, have regular follow-ups, and promptly report any health changes to their doctor. With proper care and monitoring, many patients can still have successful kidney transplants and lead healthier lives.

The key is to catch any signs of recurrence early to protect the transplanted kidney's function.

Factors that increase the risk of lupus returning in kidney transplant recipients (figure 5):

Risk factors for the Lupus recurrence in the transplanted kidney
1. African American patients
2. Female gender
3. Younger age
4. More aggressive disease in the native kidneys

Figure 5: Risk factors for lupus nephritis in the transplanted kidney

Both patients and kidney doctors need to understand that lupus can come back in a transplanted kidney, which may lead to complications and a higher risk of losing the kidney and even death (17). Factors like racial background, gender, age, specific autoimmune antibodies, and the type of donor can all affect the chances of lupus nephritis returning in transplant patients.

African American patients tend to face a higher chance of experiencing recurrent lupus nephritis in their transplanted kidneys, which can lead to less favorable outcomes. Studies show a connection between African American ethnicity and the recurrence of lupus nephritis, along with potentially lower survival rates after transplantation. This group might not respond as well to treatments, which can lead to quicker progression to end-stage kidney disease and serious health issues (15, 18, 19).

Young African American women with lupus nephritis who progress to end-stage kidney disease at a young age are vulnerable to a severe disease course. This group often faces intense symptoms and faster progression to kidney failure. These results underscore the importance of tailored medical interventions and increased surveillance for high-risk populations to enhance their success post-transplant. Medical providers should diligently identify these risk factors and deliver holistic care to address lupus nephritis recurrence in transplanted kidneys to improve survival rates and quality of life for these individuals (15).

Recurrence of lupus nephritis after kidney transplant is common in younger patients. Younger patients often face severe types of lupus nephritis. This might be due to a more active immune response and the absence of certain health issues that older individuals may have. As a result, managing lupus nephritis in younger patients usually calls for closer monitoring and a more proactive treatment strategy to help reduce the risk of recurrence.

Additionally, women face a greater risk of recurrent lupus nephritis. This heightened risk is influenced by hormonal and genetic factors that can affect how the immune system functions in women. Given that lupus primarily impacts women, especially those in their childbearing years, healthcare providers need to understand the specific challenges in this group. The cyclical hormonal changes that occur during menstruation and pregnancy can worsen lupus symptoms and may play a role in the recurrence of kidney disease.

Managing and treating recurrent lupus nephritis in the transplanted kidney

To confirm a diagnosis of recurrent lupus nephritis in a transplanted kidney, doctors typically need to perform a kidney biopsy and examine kidney tissue under a microscope. This procedure allows them to identify specific changes in the kidney associated with lupus nephritis and to rule out rejection in the transplanted kidney. While blood tests measuring complement levels and anti-double-stranded DNA antibodies are commonly used to monitor lupus, they are ineffective in diagnosing lupus nephritis in a transplanted kidney. The biopsy is essential for obtaining accurate information to guide treatment decisions.

The treatment for recurrent lupus nephritis in a transplanted kidney varies based on the severity of the condition. For milder cases, known as Class I or II lupus nephritis, improving blood pressure control is often sufficient to manage the condition. Ensuring well-controlled blood pressure can help reduce kidney strain and prevent further complications.

However, when lupus nephritis is more severe, it may require changes to the immunosuppressive medications. Adjusting these medications can help better control the lupus activity, but it also means that patients need to be monitored closely for potential side effects. This includes being vigilant about the risk of infections and cancers, which can increase due to immunosuppressive therapy. Regular check-ups and careful observation are essential to catch any issues early and ensure the best possible outcome for the patient (20).

Outcomes after transplantation

The likelihood of losing a kidney transplant due to recurrent lupus nephritis is relatively low, which is excellent news for many patients who have kidney failure from lupus nephritis. Research indicates that this risk is under 2 to 4 percent over a span of 5 to 10 years (21, 22). This is encouraging because it shows that kidney transplants can be quite successful for those who have experienced lupus nephritis. One reason for this positive outcome is that many individuals notice a reduction in lupus activity after reaching end-stage kidney disease. This means that the inflammation and damage from lupus in the kidneys often lessen when patients are preparing for a kidney transplant.

Most patients who experience recurrent lupus nephritis post-transplant tend to have milder forms of kidney disease. With only mild kidney issues, patients may have a better chance of keeping their transplanted kidney functioning well and enjoying a healthier life afterward.

However, it's important to acknowledge that some transplant patients may still encounter challenges. Many of these individuals could face issues due to other underlying factors, such as acute rejection, chronic allograft nephropathy, or medication nephrotoxicity. Acute rejection occurs when the immune system mistakenly attacks the new kidney, while chronic allograft nephropathy is a long-term concern affecting the kidney's function over time. Calcineurin inhibitors, which help prevent rejection, can sometimes lead to side effects that negatively impact kidney function. Therefore, healthcare teams must closely monitor transplant patients, ensuring any complications are quickly identified and managed.

In short, while the risk of losing a kidney transplant due to recurrent lupus nephritis is relatively low, ongoing care and monitoring are key to maintaining kidney health. Patients are encouraged to actively engage with their healthcare providers, ask questions, and discuss health or treatment concerns. By understanding the various types of kidney issues, recognizing potential symptoms, and sticking to prescribed medications, patients can help safeguard their transplanted kidneys. This proactive approach empowers patients to take control of their health and enhances their overall quality of life after a kidney transplant.

Conclusion

Kidney transplantation offers new hope for patients with lupus nephritis who progress to kidney failure. While the journey involves careful evaluation, ongoing monitoring, and lifelong medications, the benefits can be life-changing — improved health, freedom from dialysis, and a better quality of life. Although lupus nephritis can return in a transplanted kidney, this risk is relatively low with modern treatments and vigilant follow-up. Success depends on early planning, strong partnerships with the healthcare team, and personalized care that addresses both lupus and kidney health.

Take home points

- A kidney transplant is the best form of kidney replacement therapy in patients with kidney failure from lupus nephritis.
- The pre-transplant evaluation process involves extensive assessments, highlighting the need for patience and resilience.
- Ongoing monitoring and management after transplantation are vital for the health of the new kidney and overall well-being.
- There is a risk of recurrence of lupus nephritis in the transplanted kidney, which can increase the risk of allograft loss. Hence, close monitoring for lupus activity is needed after a kidney transplant.

References

1. Goo YS, Park HC, Choi HY, Kim BS, Park YB, Lee SK, et al. The evolution of lupus activity among patients with end-stage renal disease secondary to lupus nephritis. Yonsei Med J. 2004;45(2):199-206.
2. Kobayashi M, Iitsuka T, Ishizu T, Hirayama K, Igarashi M, Yamaguchi N, et al. Clinicopathological study of dialysis patients with lupus nephritis. Nihon Jinzo Gakkai Shi. 1995;37(8):456-61.
3. Pahl MV, Vaziri ND, Saiki JK, Upham T, Ness R. Chronic hemodialysis in end-stage lupus nephritis: changes of clinical and serological activities. Artif Organs. 1984;8(4):423-8.
4. Correia P, Cameron JS, Ogg CS, Williams DG, Bewick M, Hicks JA. End-stage renal failure in systemic lupus erythematosus with nephritis. Clin Nephrol. 1984;22(6):293-302.
5. Gaillard F, Bachelet D, Couchoud C, Laouenan C, Peoc'h K, Simon Q, et al. Lupus activity and outcomes in lupus patients undergoing maintenance dialysis. Rheumatology (Oxford). 2024;63(3):780-6.

6. Krane NK, Burjak K, Archie M, O'Donovan R. Persistent lupus activity in end-stage renal disease. Am J Kidney Dis. 1999;33(5):872-9.
7. Cheigh JS, Stenzel KH. End-stage renal disease in systemic lupus erythematosus. Am J Kidney Dis. 1993;21(1):2-8.
8. Ponticelli C, Moroni G. Renal transplantation in lupus nephritis. Lupus. 2005;14(1):95-8.
9. Bumgardner GL, Mauer SM, Payne W, Dunn DL, Sutherland DE, Fryd DS, et al. Single-center 1-15-year results of renal transplantation in patients with systemic lupus erythematosus. Transplantation. 1988;46(5):703-9.
10. Yap KS, Urowitz MB, Mahood Q, Medina-Rosas J, Sabapathy A, Lawson D, et al. The utility of lupus serology in predicting outcomes of renal transplantation in lupus patients: Systematic literature review and analysis of the Toronto lupus cohort. Semin Arthritis Rheum. 2017;46(6):791-7.
11. Naveed A, Nilubol C, Melancon JK, Girlanda R, Johnson L, Javaid B. Preemptive kidney transplantation in systemic lupus erythematosus. Transplant Proc. 2011;43(10):3713-4.
12. Stone JH, Amend WJ, Criswell LA. Outcome of renal transplantation in ninety-seven cyclosporine-era patients with systemic lupus erythematosus and matched controls. Arthritis Rheum. 1998;41(8):1438-45.
13. Oliveira CS, d Oliveira I, Bacchiega AB, Klumb EM, Albuquerque EM, Souza E, et al. Renal transplantation in lupus nephritis: a Brazilian cohort. Lupus. 2012;21(5):570-4.
14. Norby GE, Strom EH, Midtvedt K, Hartmann A, Gilboe IM, Leivestad T, et al. Recurrent lupus nephritis after kidney transplantation: a surveillance biopsy study. Ann Rheum Dis. 2010;69(8):1484-7.
15. Contreras G, Mattiazzi A, Guerra G, Ortega LM, Tozman EC, Li H, et al. Recurrence of lupus nephritis after kidney transplantation. J Am Soc Nephrol. 2010;21(7):1200-7.
16. Burgos PI, Perkins EL, Pons-Estel GJ, Kendrick SA, Liu JM, Kendrick WT, et al. Risk factors and impact of recurrent lupus nephritis in patients with systemic lupus erythematosus undergoing renal transplantation: data from a single US institution. Arthritis Rheum. 2009;60(9):2757-66.
17. Pattanaik D, Green J, Talwar M, Molnar M. Relapse and Outcome of Lupus Nephritis After Renal Transplantation in the Modern Immunosuppressive Era. Cureus. 2022;14(1):e20863.

18. Enfrein A, Pirson V, Le Guern V, Karras A, Tamirou F, Costedoat-Chalumeau N, et al. Worse long-term renal outcome of lupus nephritis patients of African descent living in Europe. RMD Open. 2022;8(2).
19. Lea JP. Lupus nephritis in African Americans. Am J Med Sci. 2002;323(2):85-9.
20. Wilhelmus S, Bajema IM, Bertsias GK, Boumpas DT, Gordon C, Lightstone L, et al. Lupus nephritis management guidelines compared. Nephrol Dial Transplant. 2016;31(6):904-13.
21. Goral S, Ynares C, Shappell SB, Snyder S, Feurer ID, Kazancioglu R, et al. Recurrent lupus nephritis in renal transplant recipients revisited: it is not rare. Transplantation. 2003;75(5):651-6.
22. Clark WF, Jevnikar AM. Renal transplantation for end-stage renal disease caused by systemic lupus erythematosus nephritis. Semin Nephrol. 1999;19(1):77-85.